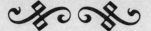

CARLTON FREDERICKS' PROGRAM FOR LIVING LONGER

by

Carlton Fredericks, Ph.D.

A FIRESIDE BOOK

Published by Simon and Schuster

NEW YORK

A Fireside Book
Published by Simon & Schuster
A Division of Gulf & Western Corporation
Simon & Schuster Building
Rockefeller Center
1230 Avenue of the Americas
New York, New York 10020

FIRESIDE and colophon are registered trademarks of Simon & Schuster.

Designed by Stanley S. Drate

Manufactured in the United States of America

Printed and bound by Fairfield Graphics

2 4 6 8 10 9 7 5 3

Library of Congress Cataloging in Publication Data

Fredericks, Carlton.
Carlton Fredericks' Program for living longer.
"A Fireside book."
Includes index.
1. Longevity—Nutritional aspects. 2. Aging—
Nutritional aspects. I. Title.
QP85.F73   1983   613.2   83-343

ISBN: 0-671-47237-2

To my beloved wife.
She taught me to try to meet
the needs of others
with understanding and compassion.
I dedicate this book to my Betty.

CONTENTS

CARLTON FREDERICKS' PROGRAM FOR LIVING LONGER

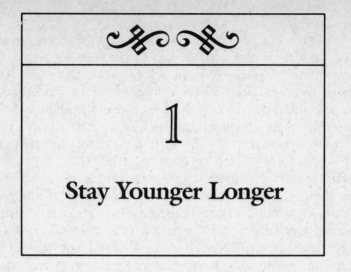

1

Stay Younger Longer

We begin to age the day we're born, which means that the time to slow the process—and we *can* slow it—is now. For young adults, the information in this book can prolong the prime of life. For you who are middle-aged, it can help to slow or even reverse some of the physical and mental deterioration that comes with time. And for those who are falling behind in the race with the calendar, what you are about to read offers genuine hope for avoiding senility or reversing it, and escaping the nursing home.

To use what we already know about anti-aging factors requires an understanding not only of their identity and actions, but also of the dietary errors that deprive us of their help. Even before you set out to understand the failures in your own nutrition, you must change you attitude toward the clock and the calendar. You must realize that time is but a yardstick, measuring duration. A ruler measures but causes nothing, and in the case of the calendar, that includes aging. You blame gray hair on old age, yet there are twelve-year-old children with gray hair. You excuse your arthritis as one of the disabilities that come with old age, but there are arthritic children, and there are oldsters whose joints are free of pain and stiffness. Perhaps the example that best brings the philosophy home is the strange pituitary disorder known as progeria, in which a child ages twenty years for each of his birthdays, so that he may perish—literally, of senility—before he is six years old.

This implies that there is an internal clock in our bodies, and indeed there is. Women who have mentally skipped birthdays can't fool the body when it is time for menopause, for example. But there is another mechanism, built into the cells, that calls a halt at a predetermined point. Research at the Wistar Institute in Philadelphia, though predictably disputed by other scientists, indicates that our cells are able to reproduce only about fifty times. When you reach the end of the line, in cells important to the pituitary, the brain, or the heart, the results are disastrous. This sounds as if we are in the position of the sorcerer's apprentice, using a whiskbroom to try to stem a cataract of woes. Actually, if the theory is correct, and we are limited in the number of generations of cells, the *rate* at which they die will certainly be affected by both life-style and diet.*

If you associate aging with feebleness, degenerative disease, wrinkling, and blunting of mental acuity, consider that I write these lines as I approach my seventy-second birthday, and this is my fourteenth book, twelve of them written after I was fifty years of age, in hours wrested from a relentless (and still continuing) schedule of broadcasts, some forty thousand of them in forty years, and teaching at universities and medical schools and societies, lecturing to the public, and supervising nutritional therapies for the professions.

The skeptical will ask about heredity, because it is convenient to credit the genes as dominant in determining the rate at which you age. Certainly, it's helpful if you are astute enough to pick long-lived ancestors with a gift for remaining youthful, but there are many—myself included—who are proof that although good heredity helps,

---

*The addition of vitamin A to a culture medium adequate for the growth of human skin cells resulted in additional generations of the cells, beyond the usual limit. This experiment, taking place *in vitro,* suggests but doesn't prove that an optimal intake of the vitamin may allow our skin to evade the built-in limits on cell regeneration.

it isn't essential. For example, the men in my family aged quickly, and many of them died relatively young.

Given my forty-plus years in the fields of public health and nutrition, it is reasonable to assume that my life-style and food choices played a part in slowing aging. This is partially so, but it isn't the whole story. It is true that if I wanted to age laboratory animals prematurely, I'd feed them as average Americans feed themselves. That would include overeating, excessive amounts of processed starches and sugars, and nutritional deficiencies, constituting a perfect formula for making the animals' internal clocks run abnormally fast.

Behavioral psychologists would ask whether I completely discount psychological factors, like stress, with malign influences on the body. The term "stress" has unfortunately been associated with destructive, negative influences that should be avoided or at all costs mitigated. Behind this are two misconceptions that you must discard if this book is to help you. Without stress, man is likely to be less productive, and attitudes toward stress are physiologically more important than the pressures on which they are focused. Consider the implications of the old joke in which the husband finds his wife in the arms of his friend. "*I* must," he protests, "but *you*?" The moral: one man's stress is another man's mistress. The unendurable for me may be a constructive stimulus for you.

There is another aspect of stress, to which a distinguished physician, Dr. Paul Rosch, has repeatedly pointed. He cites the long life spans, the vigorous good health in very old age, and the retention of the characteristics of youth by those who work in highly stressed occupations, but who are good at what they do, enjoy doing it, and are acclaimed in their fields—conductors of symphony orchestras, for instance, many of whom are still on the podium in their eighties and even nineties.

There are forty-year-olds who are physiologically sixty and seventy-year-olds who are young. Moreover, aging may be and often is selective in the organs it targets. One may have young eyes and old skin, old kidneys and a young heart. But, just as it is possible to target nutrition to slow aging, so can it be framed to help relieve the burden on a failing organ. That includes the brain: failure of memory, shortening of the concentration span, paranoid thinking, irritability, and asocial behavior are easily blamed on "old-timer's disease," but many are mistakenly labeled "senile dements" for symptoms caused by what I call the Terrible *D*'s. These are:

> Depression
> Dietary deficiency
> Dehydration
> Disease
> Drugs
> Disturbances of glands
> Desertion
> Deafness

(If deafness as a cause of supposedly senile behavior puzzles you, you are not alone. Few families may realize that the seemingly paranoid thinking of the hard-of-hearing often comes from their belief that the conversations they can't hear are whispered criticisms of *them*.)

A few case histories will illustrate how some of the Terrible *D*'s can be overlooked as underlying causes of purported senility. In the first, a woman was recently widowed, after fifty years of marriage. Her husband gone, her sons married and out of the nest, she found no interest in preparing meals, and her diet degenerated. Ultimately, she became paranoid, believing her sons to be strangers who were bent on poisoning her. She spoke daily of her wish for death. Her walk became a shuffle, with her head down, as if she were watching each step, reflecting her short perspective on life. A psychiatrist pronounced her senile and recommended a nursing home. In this the family physician concurred, diagnosing atherosclerosis (hardening of the arteries) of the brain. He, too, suggested sending her to a nursing home, since her sons could not provide for the constant nursing care she needed. I was consulted as the port of last resort—a familiar role for the nutritionist. I suggested an examination by another physician, and recommended an elderly practitioner, for the good reason that I have found them more interested in geriatric medicine than younger physicians usually are. He arrived at the same diagnosis, but I challenged it, pointing out the likelihood of the empty-nest syndrome, with hasty snacks instead of nourishing meals. I also used a Wood light to demonstrate, as ordinary light might not, that her tongue was abnormally bare, shiny, and magenta in color. At the corner of her mouth were cracks running parallel with the lips. These can be caused by ill-fitting false teeth, but, coupled with the magenta tongue, they strongly suggested a dietary deficiency. Ultimately, she was treated for what she actually suffered: the early stages of pellagra, a dietary deficiency disease in which there are mental disturbances, up to and often including outright psychosis. When last I saw her, she walked vigorously with head held high, and this reflected the change in her mental perspective on life, for she was making plans for her summer vacation.

A deficiency in a metal and a vitamin was the unrecognized cause of pseudosenility in another aged patient. He, too, had lost his mate after many years of marriage. Such a loss in men is more threatening than it is in women, for their immune systems weaken, and they fall prey to cataclysmic diseases, usually in a year or two after the wives' deaths. The patient showed symptoms in the skin, eyes, tongue, and lips that were clearly indicative of dietary deficiency. He was an affluent man who had a maid to cook his meals, so it was hard to decide why he was a victim of malnourishment. Ultimately, we discovered that a deficiency in zinc and vitamin A had distorted his sense of taste, so that familiar foods tasted rancid. This was the path into dietary deficiencies which were multiple, for he literally gagged when he tried to eat. After his diet was rectified, and supplemented with zinc and vitamin A, the derangement of the sense of taste faded gradually away. Had it not been for patient testing by the medical nutritionist on the case, the doors of the nursing home would have yawned wide for him. And in the nursing home, do you think his distaste for food would have been neatly catalogued as one of the vagaries of the aged?

Another history is that of a ninety-four-year-old attorney whom I encountered when I visited a nursing home. As I entered the home, I noticed the aged lawyer, who sat all day in an easy chair, facing the outer door, his eyes unfocused and his attention somewhere else. I improved the menus in the home, and returned some six months later, to find that improve nutrition had strikingly benefited some of the patients, and the addition of a vitamin B complex supplement to the daily diet had eliminated the "laxative line" at the pharmacy every morning. But it was the elderly lawyer who made that visit memorable. He was still in his easy chair, but he was reading the *New York Times*.

A friend called me, emotionally bankrupt with what appeared

to be senility, out of the blue, in her seventy-year-old husband. The diagnosis was, of course, cerebral atherosclerosis. I accepted that, but suggested that she take him to a medical nutritionist for chelation, a treatment that often removes the plaques from the arteries and significantly improves circulation. The physician performed the chelation, but called me to tell me that the patient's troubles included a highly overactive thyroid gland which was responsible for many of his symptoms. Once again, it had been overlooked because the diagnosis of senility seems so logical when the patient is old and his mental faculties are impaired.

Although I, as a lay nutritionist, have not had the opportunity personally to observe it, many physicians have treated patients mistakenly diagnosed as senile who were actually suffering from overdoses of a drug or from interactions among several drugs simultaneously prescribed. A typical example was a man with heart disease, for which digitalis was prescribed. The dose of this drug is critical, for a blood level that is effective must be achieved but not exceeded; overdoses can be dangerous. When this patient was fifty-five, the prescribed amount of digitalis was suited to his need, but when he reached seventy, that need had changed. He was now fifteen pounds lighter, and weight is a factor in determining the drug dose required; and he was now fifteen years older, bringing him to an age when drugs are metabolized more slowly. (It is said that each added year adds one hour to the time the body takes to inactivate and excrete a drug.) He narrowly escaped being institutionalized with a diagnosis of senility. Fortunately, his behavior returned to normal when his digitalis prescription was adjusted to his weight and slowed metabolism.

I have told you enough to indicate our resources for (and my sympathy for) those erroneously tagged with the label of "old-timer's disease." But perhaps, in the carefree way of those who believe that all the dreadful things happen to someone else, you are impatient with this prolonged discussion of real and pseudosenility. Don't be. There is an axiom in nutrition that you should commit to memory: what nutrition cures or helps, it usually prevents or mitigates. What reverses senility, then, can be applied *preventively*. That is the great virtue of scientific nutrition as compared with medical therapies. You obviously can't take digitalis today for the heart disease of tomorrow.

The goal in this book is obviously not survival alone, but putting more life into the years that ordinarily are signposts on a downward path. And that doesn't mean munching on carrot sticks and raisins. I am reminded of the time I was dining with Bob Cummings, long-time star of motion pictures and television, and two women in the restaurant recognized both of us (I still don't know how they knew *him*). One of them commented, "Both of those men are over sixty." Her companion surveyed us critically and said, "They don't look it." "Why should they," was the response, "when both of them are health nuts?" One doesn't have to be a health nut to take intelligent advantage of all the factors that help to retard aging, sometimes to reverse it, and frequently to mitigate or eliminate the penalties that come with it.

The prophylaxis suggested by successful therapy is beautifully illustrated in the progress we in nutrition have made with what I call "psychonutrition." The term is defined in a book that I wrote long ago. I said: "The term 'molecules of madness' is carefully chosen, for whether the psychosis is gene-dictated, or the price of intolerable strain, or the direct result of a derangement of the exquisitely concatenated chemistries of the brain and nervous system, in the end, the mental sickness is a molecular disease, or it is not a disease at all." When senility is appraised from that point of view, it sometimes becomes treatable, and the responses range from the slight to the dramatic. Every such response in the mentally crippled elderly demonstrates not only the possibility of preventing such disorders in the aged, but also that of improving mental function in younger, normal adults. And that isn't theory. We've done it.

Typical is the seventy-year-old who exasperates and worries the family because she remembers in minute detail what happened forty years ago, but can't find her way home from the grocery store. Medical doctrine long had it that failure of short-term memory simply means that the slate of the brain is filled with information from long ago, and there is simply no room for recent memories. It is a persuasive theory, until you think about the eighty-year-olds whose full lives have crammed innumerable long-term memories into their brains, and yet left adequate room for more recent information. The theory disintegrated when we discovered that many of these confused aged have a deficiency of acetylcholine, which is a brain compound important to memory processes. There are numerous such "neurotransmitters," which in the soggy computer of the brain are the equivalent of the wires that link the microchips in a computer. We have learned, so long ago that the lag in applying it is frustrating, that one doesn't have to surrender to a deficiency in acetylcholine. We can encourage the brain to manufacture more of it. And, again, I am not voicing theory. Inducing increased synthesis of acetylcholine by means of harmless nutrients has been used to improve short-term memory, and not only in the aged and senile, but even in young, normal individuals.

Another neurotransmitter that is synthesized in the body from dietary precursors is serotonin. Encouraging that chemistry has lifted depression, even in the suicidal, a boon as useful to the young as it is to the depressed oldster. While our knowledge of these chemistries is scanty, we do know enough to help not only the senile, but also those who don't want to surrender to time as a warper of emotions and a thief of mental functions.

An astonishingly small deficit in an essential nutrient—that is, one the body can't manufacture for itself—can twist your emotions, age you prematurely, or create or worsen symptoms of senility. Take an almost universal American (and British) dietary habit: a comforting cup of hot tea. In it there is tannin, which has the capacity to trap thiamine (vitamin B_1). There are many, young and old, whose diets yield a marginal supply of this nutrient, and interference with its availability becomes then an added insult which may be the last straw. A chronic mild deficiency of thiamine won't cause beri-beri, but it can trigger asocial behavior in teenagers and in adults; in the aged, that symptom will promptly be blamed on old age itself. Thiamine deficiency can cause difficulties with concentration and memory, accepted in younger people as a "normal" handicap, but misinterpreted in the aged as the mental price for living too long.

With protein foods the most costly on the menu, and the budgets of the elderly limited, not only is protein deficiency created, but a concomitant lack of niacinamide, which the body not only obtains, preformed, from food, but manufactures from a protein acid. This deficiency contributes to painful joints, again easily blamed on aging, and to disturbances of sleep, mental function, and total personality.

The mention of niacinamide brings up an interesting example of the lesson in prevention that arises from successful therapy with nutrients. Osteoarthritis, long linked with the wear and tear of the aging process, and common in elderly people, has successfully been treated with this vitamin, but niacinamide taken early enough can also help to prevent the disease. That is not theory; individuals who have maintained a high intake of this vitamin have not only avoided osteoarthritis, but have maintained normal joint mobility well into advanced age.

There are cosmetic dividends from sane nutrition, too. Gray hair may appear in well-fed individuals, but later than usual, and there are instances in which good nutrition has recolored gray hair. It also has helped to retain subcutaneous fat, thus avoiding or minimizing the wrinkles universally accepted as inevitable with time. There are nutrients specifically important to muscle tone. Their use, coupled with programs of exercise gaited to the individual's needs and tolerance, has resulted in reversal of the physiological clock, which translates as muscular performance reverted to that considered normal for individuals twenty years younger. The cultural lag between discovery and acceptance and application is well illustrated here: the effect of this nutrient on muscle tone was recognized thirty years ago, yet it has been neglected to this day.

You have, in reading this book, embarked on a journey of discovery that will yield dividends, whether you are interested in the welfare of an aging friend or relative or in helping yourself to stay younger longer.

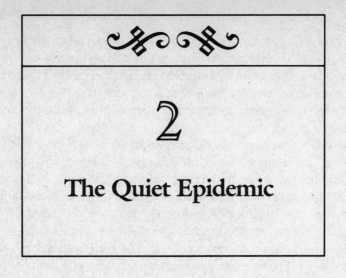

2

The Quiet Epidemic

A physician described to me how the wife of a senile seventy-five-year-old stormed into the office of her husband's geriatrician, who was expecting to be congratulated on the success of medication, hyperbaric oxygen, and nutritional therapy in restoring the patient to the world of reality and enabling him to return home. Instead, the wife declared indignantly: "He just asked me about the savings and checking accounts, what's going on in the business, and details he hasn't even thought about for years. Whatever you're doing, stop it!"

Guilt is the usual feeling of families compelled to surrender to the realities of senility and the constant care it requires, which is perhaps available to the rich in their homes, but for the rest of us, only in a nursing home. Most families have come to realize, though, that however competent the nursing and medical staffs and however pleasant the surroundings, these establishments offer only custodial care, not rehabilitation. Moreover, the removal to a strange environment is of itself a devastating change for the aged; less so if they are not in touch with reality, but even then, a negative influence. The pity of it is that although diagnosis may be accurate, the condition is not recognized as treatable. Still greater a tragedy is the percentage of diagnoses that are far off target. To that subject, this chapter is devoted.

Medical studies have shown that a significant percentage of "senile dements" committed to nursing homes and institutions actually have unrecognized and reversible *physical* disorders, which, obviously, go untreated. We are often startled by the action of mind on body, but the pendulum has swung so far that we often forget the influence of body on mind.

Filed at the University of Texas is a Ph.D. thesis recording the results of careful *physical* examination of a large number of patients committed to psychiatric hospitals for "mental" diseases, whose actual illnesses were physical rather than primarily psychiatric. A similar study was made of 136 elderly patients in nine nursing homes. Extensive neurological examinations were done, in some cases backed up with X-ray scans of the brain and electroencephalograms (EEGs), or tracings of brain waves. Complete blood chemistries were performed. The patients, 111 of them, submitted to these searching examinations included 59 with untreatable (or at least essentially irreversible) disorders, such as physical degeneration of the brain (Alzheimer's disease) or dementia as a result of blood clots from repeated strokes. Twenty-six patients had a group of such disorders as partial causes of their behavioral problems, but they also suffered from other complicating (and treatable) abnormalities, such as underactive thyroids or low blood levels of vitamin B_{12}. This, of course, opened the possibility of improving their condition by appropriate treatment. It is the third group that is tragic: twenty-six patients with treatable clinical problems ranging from "water on the brain" to underactive thyroids, low levels of vitamin B_{12}, or depression masquerading as senility. This last group could escape the snake pit, but, given custodial care rather than appropriate treatment, will remain there.

One cannot say that the same percentage of treatable disorders behind seeming senility would appear in other nursing home populations, but you can be sure that *some* patients in virtually every institution for the aged do not belong there. I am well aware that it would be cruel to give false hope to the families of the senile, but you will agree that it is at least equally cruel to label as senile a person who actually has a treatable physical disorder which is responsible for the symptoms labeled mental.

As I write about these problems, there is at the back of my mind an incident that long has haunted me. In my professional capacity as a nutritionist, I visited a nursing home where, in a small room, I found an aged woman spread-eagled on the bed, her wrists and ankles tied to the frame. The nurse explained, with no hint of apology, "She is confused and gets into trouble if we let her wander around." Translation: our staff is too small to give her proper attention. I find comfort in the thought that I have seen but this one example of professional bankruptcy of this kind; still, you will understand that I left that room with the determination to do everything possible to keep the elderly in the care of loving families, and what you are reading is part of that effort.

There is genuine hope for sufferers of the very long list of medically recognized *reversible* causes of senile behavior. Depression leads the list. The aged survivor in a long-term marriage is not only overwhelmed by melancholy, but plagued by feelings of guilt. It isn't rational to ask "Why am I the survivor?" but emotion isn't logical, and the total impact is devastating, for it parrots the symptoms of old-timer's disease, and yet yields to treatment. Moreover, that treatment need not make a zombie of the elderly patient with mind-bending antidepression drugs, for there are nutritional therapies for depression and anxiety, discussed later in this text.

The wary physician knows that depression may be the pathway to secret alcoholism, into which some of the elderly slip when seeking a shield against unbearable realities. There is also drug addiction, facilitated by the busy physician's failure to keep an eye on the patient's prescription record. The same omission is sometimes responsible for the malign effects of prescribed medication, because of either overuse, overdose, or improper mixes of drugs. Sometimes the patient, inadvertently or deliberately, does not tell the physician that he or she is visiting other doctors who are also prescribing medications; not infrequently, the pharmacist, if the patient patronizes only one drugstore, must sound the alarm.

Poisoning with heavy metals can be the culprit in some cases. Lead poisoning is usually discussed as a threat to children, because they are so sensitive to this metal, but it is more of a threat to the elderly—with their lifetime accumulation of it—than the public realizes. Cadmium is another offender, though it is more likely to cause hypertension than mental disturbances. Aluminum poisoning, tentatively blamed for the actual degeneration of nerves in the brain, can cause a type of senility that appears to come out of the blue, sometimes in startlingly young sufferers. This, unlike lead poisoning, has been regarded as untreatable, a gloomy view with which some nutritionists, including me, would disagree. Of this, more later.

The aged can show a remarkable tolerance for physiological insults that younger people would find unbearable. As an example, "silent gallstones" are found in senior citizens who never had a gallbladder attack or showed intolerance for fats, spices, and roughage. However, interference with the oxygen supply can become an intolerable burden for the aged heart and brain. Exposure to carbon monoxide, for instance, might initiate or aggravate seeming senility.

There are many disturbances of body chemistry and of the glandular system that are treatable, and to the extent that they respond, so may the purported dementia of the senile. These include kidney failure, deficiency in sodium (salt), low blood sugar, liver failure, an underactive or overactive thyroid, excessively elevated blood calcium, adrenal failure, and underactivity of the pituitary gland.

There are physical ills of the brain that can cause changes in behavior. Strokes, of course, are among these. Resulting blood clots in the brain can work mischief, and often the process is dismissed as the capriciousness of an aged mind. Yet changes in personality—untidiness in an individual who was formerly neat, or pursuit of young women by an aged man who previously had not played Don Juan—can originate with small strokes, without the gross physical effects one associates with that term, such as paralysis or speech difficulties. Sometimes surgery can be the trigger for changed behavior, which in some cases results from small strokes following an operation. Even when the complication of such strokes is not present, the aged person who undergoes surgery may develop what doctors call an "acute confusional state." It is brought on by dehydration, by lack of oxygen, by low blood pressure, either caused by the surgery or preceding and being exacerbated by it. The strong sedatives administered before surgery, coupled with anesthesia and postoperative medications, can initiate a confusional state even in a young, healthy person, but the symptoms in the elderly may be misinterpreted as senility, and some patients may actually be relegated to institutions.

Tumors, benign or malignant, can alter behavior. So can infections of the brain; thus, altered personality and mental function can follow influenza, to which the aged are highly susceptible. In one instance the infection causes brain inflammation, or encephalitis. Another postinfluenza effect on the brain, less well recognized than encephalitis, is deep (even suicidal) depression. Excessive fluid in the brain, even though the pressure is normal, can alter personality. In many cases, these conditions are treatable, and some patients will improve with nutritional therapies.

Diseases affecting the heart or lungs can warp behavior. Congestive heart failure, disturbances of heart rhythm, and emphysema are examples. Although with present knowledge there are limits on the possible benefits of treatment, the aged obviously deserve the trial.

Yeast infections, such as those caused by *Candida albicans,* are more frequent than has been realized, and are not given their due as contributors to allergic reactions that may involve the brain. There are other types of infection that can underlie altered behavior in the elderly, ranging from tuberculosis to the type which causes inflammation of the heart muscle itself.

In my own field, there are numerous examples of dietary deficiencies that can cause confusion, irritability, hostile behavior, disorientation, and failure of memory. Deficiencies of vitamin B_{12}, folate (folic acid), thiamine, and niacinamide are examples of dietary inadequacies that twist personality and impede brain function. Sometimes the failure is not in the diet but in its utilization. There are digestive disorders in the aged, as in the young, which interfere with absorption from the intestinal tract. Likewise, there are failures of utilization, frequently at the enzyme level, which affect the brain and personality. Though the public thinks of allergy as the bane of hayfever sufferers, there are allergic reactions that disorder brain function, causing symptoms ranging from amnesia to confusion, again presenting the risk in the aged that these disturbances will be blamed on old age itself. These reactions are all readily treatable.

I mentioned earlier that the deaf sometimes become paranoid; so may the blind. Sensory deprivations of these types are fortified by isolation, whether at home or in the hospital. What do you think is the impact of landing in intensive care, tied to strange, exotic instrumentation like an inchoate Frankenstein's monster, with only the occasional rustle of the nurse's uniform and the clicking of electronic devices to give some hope to the sufferer that he is still in the world of the living?

There are causes of senile behavior that are anything but rare and complicated. Impacted feces are an example. They can cause many symptoms, including some of those of second childhood, and the condition is so easily avoided that it is frustrating that it must be included in this discussion. It isn't only improper diet, lacking in fiber and B vitamins, that can trigger so severe a constipation. Simple dehydration can contribute, too. Most of us know that the senses of taste and smell are impaired in many of the elderly, but few are aware that the thirst mechanism may fail to notify the elderly that they are in need of water. Not only will this make constipation worse, but it can be a direct contribution to senile behavior, for reduced fluid intake "thickens" the blood, reducing its volume and further impairing circulation to the brain. This is, of course, as easily remediable as is one type of loss of the taste sense, which is directly caused by deficiency in zinc and vitamin A. Insufficient intake of these factors by the elderly is common, and zinc is best supplied by animal protein, which is expensive, and vitamin A by foods like liver, milk, and butter, which many people avoid because of unwarranted fear of cholesterol intake. Of this, more later, too.

It is obvious that the oxygen supply to the brain is critical in maintaining intellectual function. The other side of the coin is what happens when the genuinely senile are exposed to high oxygen levels at more than ordinary atmospheric pressure. The blood oxygen is elevated, of course, but that effect lasts only minutes, and yet the benefits may last for months. So it is that as simple and common a disorder as anemia can compromise brain function, for want of oxygen. Often, this is based on iron deficiency, but there are other types, caused, for example, by lack of folate or by poor absorption of vitamin B_{12}. Significantly, the most reliable source of vitamin B_{12} is animal protein.

On the basis of the studies I have cited, simple arithmetic will help us to decide what chance there is that old-timer's disease is the wrong diagnosis, and that a treatable condition underlies the altered personality and behavior. In the four studies in the literature, 20 percent of the senile dements had treatable diseases underlying their "second childhood." Of the 80 percent with "irreversible" causes, Alzheimer's disease was found in about 48 percent, alcoholism in more than 10 percent, and multiple blood clots, aftermaths of a series of small strokes, in about 10 percent.

Although some authoritative papers and textbooks list Alzheimer's disease, multiple strokes, and alcoholism in the elderly as essentially untreatable, practitioners of the new nutrition are less pessimistic. The aluminum concentration in the brain of Alzheimer's patients has been treated, with some success, with a chelating agent (deferoxamine) that appeared to halt, if not reverse, the deterioration in some patients. Some years ago, I evolved a nutritional therapy for brain damage that received wide publicity when it rescued some coma patients. That therapy has never been applied in Alzheimer's. It should be tried.

Counting alcoholism, whatever the age of the patient, as an untreatable cause of senile dementia is not justified either. Lack of thiamine in the alcoholic can be responsible for brain degeneration, which is, at least at early stages, treatable. If the senile alcoholic's brain and liver have not been irreversibly damaged, there are other nutritional approaches that may be fruitful. Alcoholism is not a single disease, though it is approached as such by most of the agencies in the field; and in some of its forms, even in the aged, it is distinctly treatable and sometimes curable.

Those who have had small strokes tend to suffer repetition of the disorder, with increasing impact on behavior. Predicated upon that tendency, medical nutritionists, decades ago, tested a nutritional therapy aimed at strengthening the small blood vessels that are often the target for the hemorrhages. The treated patients enjoyed a sharp reduction in the number of new strokes, as compared with their previous histories and those of untreated patients, but the report at the time fell on the deaf ears of the medical orthodoxy. One hopes that the medical people who are newly interested in nutrition will now test this therapy, and delete small strokes from the list of "untreatable" sources of senile behavior.

The optimism you found in this discussion is a product of long-term observations, not a facet of my personality. Long before the term "orthomolecular psychiatry" was originated by Dr. Linus Pauling, I had the opportunity to see what happens when corrected nutrition is pitted against senile behavior. In the first case, I was the consulting nutritionist for a dermatologist whose patient had, in addition to her skin rash, symptoms of senility, with paranoid delusions of persecution. She bought her foods in sealed boxes, at different stores each day, so as to balk the men she thought were following her, trying to kill her with drugs concealed in her food. On her fifth weekly visit to the dermatologist, she was free of her dermatitis, but she also seemed so much more normal that I queried her about the poisoners who were following her. She said she didn't see them anymore, but that they were "probably hiding around the corner" when she shopped, and that she still would not buy unprepackaged foods. A month later she came back for her final checkup, and I again asked her about the men who were following her. She replied: "What men?" That dividend came directly from the corrected diet and her supplement of the vitamin B complex.

In another case, we were faced with the problem of a suspicious, hostile, irrational, and aggressive elderly man, living with his granddaughter, who was one of my secretaries. She told me that she had no social life because her grandfather, receiving her telephone calls in her absence, hung up on all callers. She described him as living on sweets, and initially, I couldn't make any changes in his diet. I suggested to my secretary that a supplement I had formulated for a missionary organization might let us gain a little momentum, for the vitamins, minerals, wheat germ, and brewer's yeast in it were concealed in a pleasant-tasting fudgelike wafer. She followed instructions and ostentatiously hid a box of the fudge in her closet, saying nothing to her grandfather. He ate nearly a half-pound of the wafers in two days, making it fortunate that it's difficult to arrive at toxicity with most vitamins and minerals. The end of the story finds me hiring another secretary, for her grandfather, now much more normal, stopped refusing calls; her social life picked up, and she married.

Geriatric medicine is often considered unchallenging by some—usually, younger—physicians. "What can you accomplish?" is a question I've heard too many times. You will need an interested and competent medical nutritionist or geriatrician to help you to explore the categorical imperatives this chapter has proposed:

1. Be sure that reversible causes have been ruled out by really careful, comprehensive, competent examination before you surrender your aged relative to a home.

2. Be sure that nutritional appraisal has been included in that "thorough" examination. It often isn't. Medical schools that don't teach nutrition—as the majority do not—graduate physicians who minimize its importance. A good medical nutritionist's expertise is a rewarding investment.

There is a contribution *you* can make to turn the clock back for the senile, even if the senility is genuine and virtually irreversible. Few families realize that their interaction with the patient tends to make the diagnosis of senility self-fulfilling. By this I mean that *your* behavior toward the patient changes to accommodate *his,* and serves thereby to perpetuate, if not to intensify, his symptoms. Consider the implications of an experiment in a ward for the senile in a large mental hospital, housing the psychotic aged with aggressive behavior, paranoia, confusion, and incontinence of bowel and bladder. Instead of treating them like rebellious children, the staff showed afternoon movies, with socializing at tables where refreshments, including beer and pretzels, were supplied. Treated like adults and given the opportunity to socialize, the patients were benefited more than they had been by mind-bending drugs with their long lists of side effects. Some of the incontinent recaptured control of their body functions; the aggressive became more social; the paranoid lost some of their delusions.

Tender loving care is the emotional equivalent of a vitamin, but it is time to recommend it for aged adults as we long have urged it for children. It may be rewarding for you to spend a few minutes in a review of the changes in your behavior toward the patient when he became senile. Were you guilty of feedback?

There is a postscript which, however distasteful, I must add for protection of the aged. Every year, some 10,000 elderly Americans kill themselves. That means that those in the over-sixty-five group, comprising only 10 percent of the American population, are responsible for 25 percent of all suicides, and that is probably an understatement, for self-destruction can be hidden behind an unde-tected overdose of drugs, failure to take drugs essential to life, or deliberate starvation. To understand this, one must see old age for what it so often is: a loss of social roles in work, the family, and the community, with inevitable loss of income, fading of status, power, and prestige, embellished with declining health. There are the unbearable personal losses in the deaths of friends and relatives. There is the loneliness. All these are pathways to depression. Those who care will watch for the warnings, the first opportunity falling to the physician, for many suicides are preceded by a visit to the doctor. The red flags to watch for are gross changes in sleeping or eating habits, loss of weight, complaints of incessant and extreme fatigue, hypochondriacal preoccupation with functions of the body, changes in mood or behavior, and unaccustomed interest (or lack of interest) in religion. As one physician wisely remarked, this march-ing of elderly lemmings over the cliff of self-destruction will not end until society comes to value old age and its experience and knowl-edge, rather than viewing it as a curse. Until that revolution in our culture, the task of protecting the elderly begins within the family.

When it's really senile dementia, you still don't surrender, at least until you have explored all the therapeutic options open to the patient. The diagnosis ordinarily is analogous to final rites, and the family's sense of guilt is assuaged when the physician suggests that a nursing home is the only solution to the problem of the twenty-four-hour care needed by the patient with "old timer's disease." There are those who refuse to surrender; to them this discussion of alternatives is dedicated. "At least," as one devoted wife said, "I'll know I did my best for him."

The most common causes of senility are atherosclerosis of the vessels feeding the brain, and degeneration of nerve tissue, or Alzheimer's disease. Families are usually presented with these diag-noses as ending all hope, which is simply another evidence of the cultural lag in medicine, the gap between findings, their acceptance, and their application to the suffering of humanity. Given occlusion of accessible blood vessels that feed the brain, like the carotid, surgery is sometimes applicable. This, though, doesn't approach the cause, but is merely directed to the symptom, which in this case would be plaques occluding the vessel and impeding blood flow to the brain. More sensible would be a mounted attack on both symptom and cause. This is accomplished with chelation, a technique in which the physician, very slowly, introduces into the circulation an agent, a synthetic protein (EDTA), that has an affinity for minerals, including the calcium which is a large part of the obstruction of the arterial system. The treatment requires four hours per session, usually is administered three times weekly for six or eight weeks, and may subsequently, as needed, be repeated. Nuclear cardiography has been used to demonstrate the effectiveness of this therapy, and showed in a case so examined a 54 percent increase in circulation to the brain. The action of EDTA isn't confined, of course, to cerebral blood vessels, but acts generally on the arteries, bodywide, and is used thereby also to increase the flow through the coronary arteries, or to improve circulation to the legs when it is impaired, as it sometimes is in diabetics.

The chelation therapy has been erroneously described as new, dangerous, and relatively untried. These negative statements originate with ignorant physicians who have never themselves administered or watched the administration of chelation. The technique, rather than new, is over thirty years old, and is infinitely safer than bypass surgery, and in many cases at least as effective. I write dogmatically because I have been an honorary president of the Academy of Medical Preventics, which is the society devoted to medical chelation, and because I have had access to the records of some eighteen thousand patients and the results of more than a million chelation sessions.

The affinity of EDTA for minerals means, of course, that some will be removed and, since they are essential, must be replaced. Of this, the chelating physician is well aware, and the vital nutrients are actually restored while the chelating session is in progress, through the intravenous drip in which the EDTA is delivered. Some senile patients, in response to chelation and to reenforcement of their nutrition, show remarkable improvements by this modality. The effects have been increased by the use of hyperbaric oxygen, a treatment in which the patient is exposed to oxygen in a concentration and at a pressure beyond that in the air we normally breathe. By way of demonstrating how little we know, consider that the oxygen overload leaves the blood in a very short time, and yet the benefits of hyperbaric oxygen therapy have been known to persist for months.

After chelation, and after hyperbaric oxygen—less frequently used because a special tank is required—the medical nutritionist will also correct the diet, administering therapeutic doses of vitamins, minerals, protein (if needed) or amino acids, and factors, like L glutamine, which strongly stimulate the central nervous system. There are both therapeutic and prophylactic dividends from these nutritional therapies. Many cases of senility respond in varying degrees, with some restored to normalcy. Many do not respond, for nutrition has no panaceas.

Alzheimer's disease offers a bleaker prognosis. We are not even sure of the mechanism that causes nerve fibers in the brain to tangle wildly, with senility appearing, apparently overnight, making mindless vegetables of the patients, some of them shockingly young. Aluminum poisoning, concentrated in the brain, has been indicted. This is based on the one slender bit of evidence we do have: there is an abnormal concentration of aluminum in the disordered tissues of the brain in Alzheimer's disease. Conceivably, the consistency with which the accumulation of the metal is found there could be coincidence, or might be the presenting evidence of some other abnormal process, yet unrecognized. Against this, there are the observations of the response of some of these patients when they are chelated to remove aluminum. The condition isn't reversed, but its ordinarily relentless progress appears to slow or even halt. In this type of chelation, EDTA is not used, but another chelating chemical, one that originally was employed to remove excess iron from the body.

In recent years, acting on the theory that Alzheimer's disease involves a failure of the brain to produce an essential neurotransmitter, acetylcholine, in normal quantities, high phosphatidyl choline, which is a precursor of that neurotransmitter, has been employed. This agent, which is not a drug but a nutritional concentrate of a natural factor, has proved somewhat helpful in early cases of the disorder, particularly in improving the memory. In my own research in brain damage other than Alzheimer's, I have repeatedly seen improvements in patients in deep coma who were treated with a waxy alcohol, octocosanol, which is found in foods. This has rescued some coma patients with what appeared to be very severe and, by ordinary standards, irreversible brain damage, including that caused by strokes, oxygen deprivation, and carbon monoxide poisoning. I am awaiting the opportunity to observe the use of octocosanol in Alzheimer's disease. Meanwhile, the choline therapy and chelation with deferoxamine, the agent I mentioned a paragraph ago, remain the sole promising treatments actually in use.

Reference to brain damage from a stroke has reminded me of a case history, which I ask you now to read. It records the responses of a stroke victim, fortunate in having a physician with expertise in nutrition. The history is cited because strokes, both small and major, are a greased pathway into senility; drug therapy is bankrupt; prevention is possible. What you are about to read came to me directly from the courageous physician, a gynecologist. Only the names of the doctor and the patient have been omitted.

Dear Dr. Fredericks:

This is a brief history of my patient.

Two and a half years ago at the age of seventy-eight, this vivacious, intelligent 130-pound female had a mild stroke with no residual paralysis. The "best care" at a teaching center was administered, consisting of Dilantin, phenobarbital, Haldol, and other related medications. Diet and vitamins were completely neglected. This yielded a sixty-pound, anemic, cachectic, mumbling, incontinent, bedridden, disoriented vegetable. Her distraught husband was spending a fortune, and still she was dying.

On March 25, 1982, at 10 o'clock in the evening he called me and asked for help, since he felt she was expiring. She was comatose and had Cheyne-Stokes breathing. The funeral director and minister were notified. I had recently heard your broadcasts on aging and neglect of the elderly, and had taken a few notes. I rushed back to the hospital, and armed with intravenous fluids, intravenous electrolytes, glucose, vitamins, amino acids, and intravenous lipids, started treatment. Attached is my detailed list of medications.

Her response is now called a miracle. Just five months later, she is speaking coherently, answers questions appropriately, in clear, bell-like tones. She can sit up on the terrace and feed herself with grace, and she looks at magazines. The leg contractures are gradually improving, and she can pump an exercycle, and walk twenty feet with assistance. She is now having bowel movements in the bathroom. She watches television, and attempts to play cards. She is gaining weight, getting strong, struggling to get up and walk. She is taken for an automobile ride, each afternoon.

After the initial intravenous medication, we started feeding her a mixture of a protein drink with ice cream and the vitamins, blended together, fed drop by drop until now she has an appetite and is on a regular diet, plus this same protein drink with all the important vitamins. Her husband is grateful, and has permitted me to write the details to you.

The physician adds a comment that stigmatizes the cultural lag in medicine, particularly aggravated in the case of elderly patients, which largely motivated the writing of this book: "I seldom told my colleague of my faith in nutrition, for fear of the 'kook' label." In reading that, I was grimly reminded of a medical man's diary, with this comment, written in the 1890s: "I have discovered that mouldy bread is a sovereign remedy for infected throats. I have my sons in the barn, rolling the bread into pills. I shall say nothing to my colleagues, though, for fear that they would think me crazy." So the pioneer discovery of penicillin was carefully hidden, not to be disinterred for a half-century.

The physician treating the elderly lady closed with "You deserve all the credit for so diligently trying to educate physicians in spite of adverse criticism."

Appended to the letter, as promised, was the protocol of the nutritional treatment that brought this elderly patient back, literally, from the edge of the grave. While I realize that many of the nutrients used will be unfamiliar to the average reader, they are equally unfamiliar to physicians and other health care professionals who are not specialists in nutrition. The list brings up an important point; understanding it will let you cope with the indifference (if not hostility) of the profession to nutritional therapies.

INITIAL ROUTINE

Intravenous fluids:
5% Glucose
Electrolytes
B complex and vitamin C
Intravenous amino acids
Intravenous lipids

Vitamin B$_{12}$, 6,000 mcg. IM (by intramuscular injection) daily

Routine now in effect:
1. Proloid, gr. $^1/_2$
2. Niacinamide, 500 mg. 1 daily
3. Pantothenic acid, 500 mg., 1 daily
4. Taurine, 500 mg., 1 daily
5. Octocosanol, 1,000 mcg., 1 daily
6. D-glutamic acid, 500 mg., 1 daily
7. L glutathione, 50 mg., 1 daily
8. Deaner(a form of choline), 100 mg., 2 daily
9. Dolomite, 2 daily
10. Vitamin B$_{12}$, 3,000 mcg. IM 2 × weekly
11. Windswept Ultra Mega Plus, 1 daily

Vit. A, 25,000 IU	Inositol, 100 mg.
Vit. D, 1,000 IU	Niacinamide, 100 mg.
Vit. E, 150 IU (d alpha)	PABA, 100 mg.
Bioflavanoid, 30 mg.	Pantothenic Acid, 100 mg.
Vit. C, 500 mg.	Iodine, 150 mcg.
Hesperidin, 5 mg.	Zinc, 20 mg.
Rutin, 30 mg.	Manganese, 7 mg.
Vit. B$_1$, 100 mg.	Iron, 15 mg.
Vit. B$_2$, 100 mg.	Calcium, 60 mg.
Vit. B$_6$, 100 mg.	Potassium, 15 mg.
Vit. B$_{12}$, 100 mcg.	Magnesium, 40 mg.
Biotin, 100 mcg.	Chromium, 15 mg.
Choline, 100 mg.	Selenium, 50 mcg.
Folic Acid, 400 mcg.	Glutamic acid, 30 mg.
	Betaine HCL, 30 mg.

The initial reaction of the orthodox physician to this long list of nutrients will be one of, at least, skepticism and, possibly, hostility. This is likely to be predicated on a philosophy taught to all medical students: avoid polypharmacy. In other words, don't use three drugs if two will do. Not only do you run the risk of overmedication and increase the danger of side reactions, but there are interactions among drugs, and the longer the list of medications, the greater the risk of harmful interplay among them.

Applied to medications, this is perfectly true. In fact, the blunt doctor will tell you that any drug potent enough to be helpful is potent enough to have dangerous side effects, and the fewer used, the better. However, while polypharmacy is bad medical practice, it is unavoidable, necessary, and desirable in nutrition. The term "a good mixed diet" tells the story. Nutrition is a fabric of many threads. When one thread is severed, the effects reflect disturbances of the others, and treatment very frequently demands more than attention to the one thread. This is a long way of saying that polypharmacy may be bad medicine, but polynutrition is rational and necessary.

Another and more justified criticism of the protocol for this patient is the lip-service amount of some of the nutrients employed. In the quantities present in some of the formulas, some of the nutrients could not possibly have effective actions. This, however, is not the responsibility of the prescribing physician, but represents the ignorance of the manufacturers of some of the concentrates. Nonetheless, the protocol was effective, and the patient rescued, which is all that counts.

It is ironic that the medical insurance companies, hopelessly wedded to "community standards of medical practice," would probably refuse to reimburse the costs of this nutritional therapy though perfectly willing to pay for the prescriptions for phenobarbital, Dilantin, Haldol, and the other medications that allowed her to lose weight until she dropped to sixty pounds and became terminal. These lines I write by way of warning. Neither your insurance company nor your orthodox physician will desert the traditional drug therapies, however impotent they are, to help your aged patient to recover through nutritional therapies. You will, in fact, meet opposition even from the hospitals, which will cheerfully order dangerous drugs, but insist that their "new drug" committees must approve the use of a harmless vitamin.

The obstacles are obviously formidable when one is trying to protect the aged. You must be armed to cope with faulty diagnoses, and when the diagnoses are accurate and senility is really the problem, you must face the apathy with which the professions surrender to the concept that time is toxic and its effects immutable. The struggle, from what you have read, is worth the effort, if you are determined not to surrender until all possibilities have been explored.

Two important notes for those interested in prevention. The accumulation of aluminum in the brain doesn't appear out of nowhere. We are exposed to many sources of this dangerous metal, some of them unknown to you. Yes, aluminum is concentrated in deodorants, and it is entirely possible that external application permits absorption. But aluminum salts are used to clarify drinking water, are constituents of baking powder, and come to you in menacing quantities in many prescription and over-the-counter antacid drugs. Aluminum salts are also used in food additives.

The second note of prevention appears when a small stroke becomes responsible for altered and apparently senile behavior. Although such brain events are very frequent in our aged population, and sometimes astonishingly so in the younger, medicine has failed to take advantage of some of the pioneering research in the use of a nutrient to strengthen the smaller blood vessels, which are often the target for the process. Most of us know that vitamin C deficiency weakens small blood vessels, but few are aware that the bioflavonoids, which accompany vitamin C in many foods, strengthen those vessels. Some twenty years ago, a medical nutritionist applied that knowledge by giving bioflavonoid supplements to victims of little strokes. Since the process is usually ongoing, one could anticipate repeated attacks in such a group, continuing until the massive stroke, crippling if not lethal, eventuated. Those treated with the bioflavonoids became steadily more resistant to small strokes, while the control group, deprived of the supplement, suffered repeated new attacks. Citrus bioflavonoids, hesperidin, hesperidin chalcone, and rutin concentrates are all available. The citrus type is the best choice, both for effectiveness and for lower cost. In part, the citrus type is preferable because the bioflavonoids from this source are more soluble and, dissolving more readily, are better utilized. Frequently, the bioflavonoids are combined with vitamin C in supplements, but most of the formulations I've encountered are irrational in that the vitamin C potency is high and the bioflavonoid low. This reverses what nature does: a large orange may provide 100 mg. of vitamin C, but yields 900 mg. of bioflavonoids. (You discard them when you strain the juice, incidentally. So do most of the orange-juice processors.) For these reasons, I have set 3,000 mg. of bioflavonoids as the preferred daily intake.

The note on the discarding of pulp by orange-juice processors suggests that you (a) eat the whole orange and (b) never strain the juice, or (c) choose a brand of orange juice which retains some of the pulp. One other caution: orange juice in cartons is a poor choice. The loss of vitamin C is amazingly rapid. Choose glass containers.

It is perhaps startling to realize that the habits of the aging and the aged, in depriving themselves of the bioflavonoid values of fruits, may be one of the entities in the disasters we mistakenly attribute to the aging process itself. But it's true.

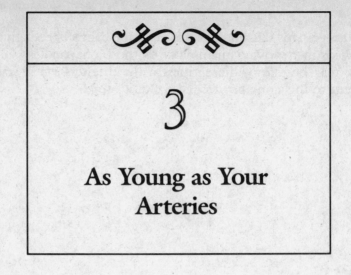

3

As Young as Your Arteries

When primitives' food choices are governed by the accumulated wisdom handed down from one generation to another, the degenerative diseases of civilization pass them by, while among us they are so common that we accept them as normal. So we learned from Central Africa natives that their freedom from constipation, diverticulitis, varicose veins, diverticulosis, and bowel cancer is a dividend from their high-fiber diet.* Still other primitives, though it took us a century to absorb the lesson, taught us that low-sodium diets prevent high blood pressure, and that it isn't normal (though with us it's average) for the pressure to rise as the years mount. The Maori mother-in-law will trudge to the seacoast, a journey that may

---

*Information on fiber to protect health and retard aging will be found in Chapter 10. For more information, see *Carlton Fredericks' High-Fiber Way to Total Health,* published by Pocket Books.

take days, to catch and dry fish to feed to her pregnant daughter-in-law. These people never heard of iodine, but somehow learned that seafood conveys something that makes for healthy mothers and babies. (Underactive thyroid glands are common in American women.)

Our orthodontists would be less affluent if we heeded what primitives know about the role of pregnancy diet, high in cooked protein, in creating infants with narrow palates who mature with crowded mouths. The yeast used to ferment the toddy favored by a primitive group was fed to nursing mothers and to babies, thereby preventing beri-beri, while the minority in our culture who take yeast as a supplement are regarded as cultists. Perhaps fortunately for our men, liberated women have not yet caught up with the herbs known to primitive peoples that allow men to lactate and take over the task of natural feeding of babies.

Barely visible on the horizon of civilized nutrition is a primitive dietary practice that may be a significant answer to our problems with atherosclerosis and heart disease. That we are struggling with an epidemic is obvious, for this year, in America alone, for 500,000 the first symptom of heart disease will be death. To that toll, add nearly another half-million Americans who will perish from strokes. Though the emphasis has been on the susceptibility of men, postmenopausal women have become increasingly vulnerable to these diseases, particularly those who smoke and those who have used the birth control pill.

The problem has not been solved by the low-cholesterol diet, nor by restrictions on animal fat intake, nor would anyone logically expect it to be. Elevated blood cholesterol and triglycerides are *risk* factors, not absolute causes of artery and heart disease. That is why there are people with elevated blood cholesterol and triglycerides who don't develop hardening of the arteries or heart disease; and those with normal or low levels who do. In fact, newborn babies, yet to make their acquaintance with eggs, butter, and liver, show the first streaks on the artery walls, portents of the atherosclerosis to come. Young soldiers killed in Korea were often found to have advanced hardening of the arteries.

Since I can't help to keep you young if your arteries are aging and growing sick, I have two obligations: (1) to teach you how to protect your blood vessels, and (2) in so doing, to keep you from unnecessary participation in a system of diet (low fat, low cholesterol, high polyunsaturated fat) that is dangerous, fails to guard your vascular system and heart, and deprives you of foods that are high in cholesterol but important to good nutrition. Hence the detailed explanations you are about to read.

There are many reasons to reject elevated blood cholesterol or triglycerides as *the* causes of atherosclerosis. In addition to those I've already described, let me add a few others:

1. A noted heart surgeon, Michael DeBakey, has remarked that he has inspected thousands of arteries and found no significant relationship between blood cholesterol levels and the conditions of the vessel walls.

2. For every country and ethnic group where high intake of fat and cholesterol is linked to artery and heart disease, you can find another where the same diet has no such effects.

3. Two-thirds of the cholesterol in the body is manufactured there. Why all the emphasis on the one-third from the diet? And why has no attention been paid to the disastrous results of attempts to lower the rate of synthesis of cholesterol with a drug?

4. Though cholesterol has become a dirty word, should not someone remind the professions and the public that it is vital to life as a precursor of a number of hormones and as the source of insulation for the nervous system?

5. Though polyunsaturated fats, principally vegetable oils, are eulogized as antidotes for cholesterol, there are countries—Israel is an example—where the diet is high in such fats, but the hospitals are nonetheless filled with patients with heart disease.

6. There is a feedback mechanism that is supposed to reduce cholesterol synthesis in the body when the dietary intake is high. The principle works beautifully in some primitives who ingest startling amounts of cholesterol but escape artery-heart disease. Why is that system not functioning as well in us?

7. How does the cholesterol theory explain the fact that heart attack rates are dramatically lower in areas where the drinking water is high in minerals (hard)? An interesting sidelight is the experience of a group of surgeons who actually witnessed the initiation of a heart attack while performing open heart surgery. It didn't involve a clot, and owed nothing to blood cholesterol. It was a spasm of the coronary vessels, clamping down on the blood supply to the heart. This could be initiated by magnesium deficiency, which has been observed in the heart tissue of many victims of heart attacks. That

would explain the linkage between soft water, which is low in magnesium, and increased incidence of such attacks.

8. The excessive emphasis on dietary cholesterol and saturated fats completely ignores the role of sugar in elevating blood fats. Although our ancestors didn't avoid fried foods, fatty gravies, and butter, they also didn't eat, as we do, what amounts to a teaspoonful of sugar every thirty-five minutes, twenty-four hours per day. Populations with high immunity to cardiac and vascular disease lose it when the "affluent" Western diet, with its tonnage of sugar, is introduced. Sugar is efficient in raising both cholesterol and triglycerides, but it is also known to increase the adhesiveness of blood cells involved in the clotting processes. This may help to damage artery walls, facilitate the formation of plaques, and contribute to coronary thrombosis. Since sugar is almost inescapable in modern food, this chapter will later give you a dietary antidote to that effect.

There are two viable theories, too long ignored, which better explain our epidemic of cardiovascular diseases. Both theories lead us to protective measures that, unlike the low-cholesterol diet, don't interfere with good nutrition and offer no possibility of harm. One of these centers on pyridoxine (vitamin B_6), a vitamin in short supply in the American diet. The other involves marine lipids (fats), which Americans largely bypass, but which appear to be protecting some primitive populations against heart and artery disease. These marine oils are provided by types of fish that Americans eat only occasionally, and they are available, fortunately, as concentrated dietary supplements.

If you want to prolong youth, and achieve an old age in which cerebral atherosclerosis does not threaten you with the nursing home, you ought to understand and profit by this research, so largely ignored by or unknown to the health professions and the public.

The homocysteine theory is complex, but it leads to a simple protection against cardiovascular diseases by increasing your intake of vitamin B_6. Since this will require a lifetime of the use of such a supplement, I am asking you to follow this biochemical trail, even if it is a bit much to inflict on nonchemists. The history begins with two young, mentally retarded sisters, whose disorder was inherited. In their urine appeared a chemical not normally found there. This, homocystine, was obviously linked in some way to atherosclerosis, for autopsies of these girls, who died in their early teens, revealed advanced hardening of the blood vessels, with the type and numbers of atherosclerotic plaques one would expect to find in the aged. These unfortunate children seemed to have concentrated into a few short years the lifetime process of atherosclerosis.

Now the chemistry: from protein foods, such as meat, fish, fowl, eggs, and most dairy products, we take our supply of amino acids, the building blocks of protein, many of which the body can't manufacture. Among these amino acids is methionine, which the body uses to make other chemicals it needs. One of these chemicals is *homocysteine*. It is toxic in excessive quantities, but in the healthy, well-nourished body, homocysteine is converted into a harmless (and necessary) chemical called *cystathionine*. This conversion necessitates the action of an adequate supply of vitamin B_6, but this vitamin, you will learn, is not available in sufficient amounts in the average American diet. In the absence of that adequate intake, the conversion into cystathionine is blocked, and the homocysteine accumulates in the body, where by the action of oxygen it is converted into *homocystine* and, in that form, reaches the urine. So much for the chemistry; now for its application to hardening of the arteries.

Alone of the B vitamins, a deficiency of vitamin B_6 causes atherosclerosis in monkeys. It was theorized that this was due to a toxic effect of the homocysteine, accumulating in the blood and attacking the delicate inner walls of the arteries. Since vitamin B_6 would have allowed the body to dispose of the homocysteine in the normal way, vitamin B_6 deficiency was linked directly to hardening of the arteries. This leads to a question: what happens when you give intravenous injections of homocysteine? In rabbits and baboons, those injections were more effective than cholesterol in causing arterial plaques, and the process of their formation is similar to that known to be behind human atherosclerosis. This led to another question: what happens to human beings deliberately fed a diet low in vitamin B_6? Does the homocysteine in their blood rise? And does this lead to excretion of the oxidized form, homocystine, in the urine? The experiments were performed, and the predictions were confirmed. A diet low in the vitamin led to elevated blood homocysteine and urinary homocystine.

These were normal subjects. What about patients with known atherosclerosis? Where were their vitamin B_6 levels? And how much homocysteine did their blood carry? Researchers in the United States and the Soviet Union reported low vitamin B_6 blood levels in such patients. These studies were done decades ago, ironically. As for the levels of homocysteine in the blood of atherosclerotic patients, it was found to be high. In the course of that research, the might-have-been-expected was also found: normal, apparently healthy people with inadequate intake of vitamin B_6 as evidenced by abnormal blood levels of homocysteine. Were these well people actually on their way to blood vessel and heart disease? And are you such a well person, lacking vitamin B_6?

Don't lose track of the nutritional components of this theory. Vitamin B_6 deficiency isn't the whole story. Remember that it is an amino acid, methionine, which is the starting point for the manufacture of homocysteine, with vitamin B_6 intervening to convert that into a nontoxic (and essential) substance, cystathionine. Therefore, the diet high in methionine becomes a threat when that diet is also low in vitamin B_6. That, unfortunately, is a description of many American diets, and note that all this has nothing to do with cholesterol or triglycerides. There is a simple fact: if you expose artery cells to homocystine, it damages them. If you want to avoid that damage, you must have in your diet a good working ratio between your intake of methionine and your intake of vitamin B_6. And thereby hangs the tale, for many, many American diets are rich in methionine and poor in the vitamin. Let us see how that happens.

If you merely survey a list of foods common in the American market basket, and appraise them for purported content of vitamin B_6 and for methionine, you would conclude that we have adequate amounts of the vitamin to help us to "handle" the amino acid. And that conclusion would be fallacious. Dairy products and meats provide generous amounts of methionine but sparse amounts of vitamin B_6. Moreover, cooking, freezing, and processing significantly deplete the vitamin B_6 content of foods. Some 40 percent of the B_6 value of meat is destroyed in cooking. The impact of food processing is drastic. Shredded wheat loses about 38 percent of its vitamin B_6. Cracked wheat bread has lost about 49 percent; puffed wheat, 56 percent; saltine crackers, 62 percent; spaghetti, about 65 percent; French bread, 70 percent; white bread, nearly 78 percent; and all-purpose flour, 82 percent. As against these losses in popular foods, consider the relative infrequency with which average Americans eat foods rich in vitamin B_6, including sunflower seeds, wheat germ, beef liver, soybeans, walnuts, salmon, chicken, bananas, halibut, and avocados.

The proponents of the cholesterol theory often point to vegetarians as "proof" that avoiding cholesterol is the key to the health of the heart and arteries. But vegetarians eat diets low in methionine and adequately supplied with vitamin B_6. Their resistance to atherosclerosis may well derive from escaping accumulation of homocysteine. These observations would also explain the fallacy in the attempts to link high-protein diets with atherosclerosis. It's not the high protein, but the low vitamin B_6 intake, linked with a generous supply of methionine. Part of the problem, then, derives from destruction of the vitamin B_6 in protein foods in high-temperature cooking, to which such foods are routinely subjected. The methionine in roast beef largely survives the high temperature; the vitamin B_6 doesn't. All this offers part of the explanation for the survival of Eskimos on diets strikingly high in fat and cholesterol, for their intake of fish and uncooked meat must provide enough vitamin B_6 to protect them. We'll return to this point, for the Eskimo has another type of protection against cardiovascular disease, contributed by a diet high in fish.

Among the many warnings given to women on the birth control pill, there is the flat statement that users may be twelve times as likely to develop blood clots and heart attacks. Interestingly, in the light of the theory we have been discussing, the pill is known to lower vitamin B_6 blood levels, which could then lead to the toxic level of homocysteine. Pregnancy, smoking, and alcoholism all increase the need for vitamin B_6.

Aside from the impact of cooking, freezing, and processing on the vitamin B_6 values of American foods, there is other evidence for widespread deficiency in this factor. Carpal tunnel syndrome, a painful disorder of the wrist, hand, and sometimes shoulder, is a common disease for which surgery is frequently performed. In the dry language of science, researchers have said: "It is not suitable to perform surgery for a condition caused by deficiency in vitamin B_6." Another group in the population who evidence a widespread deficiency in the vitamin are the women with premenstrual water retention. This condition is so common that diuretics to relieve it are advertised on television. Yet vitamin B_6 has been found to prevent it, which argues for a deficiency of the factor in millions of women. Hypertrophic arthritis is anything but a rare disease, and this disorder, too, has successfully been treated with vitamin B_6.*

Not only are there vast population groups whose intake of pyridoxine is too low, but there is reason to believe that those who achieve the recommended dietary allowance of pyridoxine could profit by more. The government recommends 2 mg. daily, and many of us don't even achieve *that*. For those of us who would like to keep our arteries young, even though we have nothing more than theory and early research to motivate us, 10 mg. daily would seem to make more sense. Among my colleagues in holistic medicine, I know a few competent medical nutritionists who would rather set 25 mg. as the goal.

Earlier, I mentioned that the Eskimos are protected by something more than a favorable methionine–vitamin B_6 ratio. That brings us to the second theory, which involves the fish oils that are a large part of the calorie intake of the Japanese, Eskimo, and other populations that don't share our problems with cardiovascular diseases, even when their diets are swimming in cholesterol and animal fats. Take a deep breath, reader: you are about to learn more about marine fatty acids than you thought you'd ever want to know. I promise that it's worth the effort, even when you must wrestle with terms like "eicosapentaenoic acid" and "docosahexaenoic acid."

To nutritionists, it is an old observation that healthy immigrants in the United States fall prey to sicknesses that were no problem in their native lands. A striking example is the Japanese woman who has high immunity to breast cancer when she lives in Japan, but who, in moving to Hawaii, ultimately becomes as susceptible as American women (of whom one in every fourteen are stricken with breast cancer). We have long known, too, that Canadian Indians and Eskimos, with access to "civilized" foods at a trading post, become susceptible to our diseases, while those remaining on their native diets retain their immunity. However, only recently was research directed to the resistance of primitives to heart and blood vessel diseases, even when their diets are high in

---

*Vitamin B_6 deficiency has been held responsible for the "Chinese restaurant syndrome," which is caused by consuming foods seasoned with large amounts of monosodium glutamate. Headache, cramps, and flushing are among reactions. Fascinatingly, many patients with carpal tunnel syndrome also suffer from Chinese restaurant syndrome.

cholesterol and animal fats. A striking observation was made by Dutch researchers, who compared the incidence of heart disease among Eskimos living in Greenland with that of Eskimos who moved to eastern Canada, where they consumed the Canadian type of diet. Within a single generation, their susceptibility to heart disease went up to the Canadian level, far above that in Greenland. Obviously, this ruled out heredity as the protection against heart disorders, and implicated a critical difference between the Greenland Eskimo diet and that consumed after the move to Canada. (The mortality rate from heart disease is 5 percent among Greenland Eskimos whose dietary staple is fish. Compare that with the 50 percent rate in Denmark!)

So much of the dietary fat of the Eskimo comes from fish that it was logical to assume that something in marine oils defends the Eskimo against heart disease. This brought the chemists into the arena, and they shortly found that there was a significant amount of an unusual fatty acid in the oils of the fish and cold-water mammals on which the Eskimos base their diet. This was eicosapentaenoic acid, which is chemically a cousin of linolenic, linoleic, and arachidonic acids.

The theory was that eicosapentaenoic acid (EPA) reduced the tendency of the blood to clot excessively. This might not only protect against a heart attack or stroke caused by a clot, but also defend the arteries against plaque formation, because excessive clotting may contribute to that, too. To understand this, you should know that there is a blood cell called a platelet, part of the normal clotting system that defends you against hemorrhage. These cells must not be too adhesive, must not clump excessively, or we become susceptible to artery-wall damage and to coronary heart attacks and strokes. (That's why I mentioned earlier the undesirable effect of sugar in increasing the stickiness of blood platelets.) Such adhesiveness and clotting can also lead to thrombophlebitis.

The research showed that the EPA in the diet is only the beginning of the story. True, examination of the blood of Greenland Eskimos showed a high concentration of this unusual fatty acid, but this was the first step in a series of chemical processes in which the body manufactures short-lived hormones call prostaglandins. Two of these, thromboxane and prostacyclin, made in the body from EPA, are the guardians which keep the platelets from abnormally sticking to each other. That, though, is only one of the dividends from EPA. It has proved to be an effective agent for reducing blood levels of both cholesterol and triglycerides, and—this is the important point—it does this most dramatically when those levels are high.

To understand the last of the proposed dividends from marine oil intake, you should backtrack now and take another look at the cholesterol theory. Cholesterol in the blood doesn't float through the vessels, seeking a break in the walls in which to deposit itself. In the body, cholesterol is neatly packaged, combined with protein, in what are called *lipoproteins*. There are a number of types of lipoproteins, all incorporating cholesterol, but only one type has the nasty habit of acting like a coal car that tips over and dumps its load. These, called low-density lipoproteins, spill their cholesterol into the blood. This property is balanced by the "high-density lipoproteins" that hang on to their cholesterol until it can be discarded where it will be excreted. Your "batting average"—meaning the ratio between your low-density and high-density lipoproteins—is obviously much more important to your health than the gross amount of cholesterol in your blood. So it is that many physicians who worshiped at the shrine of the low-cholesterol diet have quietly stopped emphasizing that. They now order tests for levels of low- and high-density lipoproteins, and regard you as protected—whatever your blood cholesterol level—if you have generous amounts of high-density and, preferably, low amounts of low-density lipoproteins. All this is relevant to our discussion of EPA, for the good reason that this marine fatty acid raises high-density lipoprotein and simultaneously lowers the level of the other type.

Which brings us to another of my favorite complaints. For many years, in lectures to the profession and the public, I have condemned the use of supplements of vitamins A and D from fish liver oil, insisting that in so processing cod liver and other fish oils, and using only the vitamins, we may be throwing the baby out with the bathwater. I have over and over again said that we have recklessly deprived babies of who-knows-what benefits by feeding them formulas—which deprive them of gamma linolenic acid—and replacing cod liver oil with vitamin A and D concentrates. I've even urged that those who visit the housebound elderly bring cod liver oil, rather than flowers or candy, for these aged people are in greater need of vitamins A and D than sweets or floral decorations. It now is certain, thanks to the research with EPA, that we *have* deprived infants and the elderly of more than we realized, for cod liver oil, as a marine oil, is a fair source of EPA. We do not propose its use for that purpose, for the reason that the dose suitable for EPA supply may yield excessive amounts of the vitamins. However, that problem has been solved, for supplements of EPA from fish oils, without the vitamins, are now available.

The medical authorities, while confessing excited interest in these findings, are curiously conservative for a profession which has freely prescribed diuretics that killed some people, and anti-inflammation drugs that were lethal to dozens of arthritics. They grant that supplements of marine oil will probably become part of our daily scheme of things that help to keep us younger and healthier; but they urge caution until we know more about the actions of these oils. Which manages to ignore completely the observation that started all the excitement: native populations consuming large amounts of oily fish and enjoying high resistance to atherosclerosis and heart disease. Aren't the Greenland Eskimos fortunate that there is no Eskimo A.M.A. to discourage their consumption of fish?

Though the high intake of oily fish in the primitive diet gives us enough assurance to justify raising our intake of EPA, there remain many exciting questions to be answered by future research. The marine oil concentrates supply significant amounts of EPA and DHA (docosahexaenoic acid, if you've forgotten). But is there some other esoteric type of fat in fish oil that contributes to the beneficial effects? Then, too, much of the testing has been done with 5 grams or more of EPA daily. This proved effective in reducing adhesiveness and the clotting tendency of the platelets, and in increasing the high-density and decreasing the low-density lipoproteins, while lowering both blood cholesterol and triglycerides. But would a smaller intake for a longer period have the same effects?

There is a question I anticipate, after discussing this subject with my university students and with the professions. Reducing the clotting tendency of platelets could be a two-edged weapon. Might it undesirably prolong the clotting time of blood, to the point where bleeding could become excessive? Not so: the clotting time is extended, but remains within normal limits.

It is interesting that, long before this research, a high-fish diet was recommended for early cases of multiple sclerosis. It has been effective in lowering the viscosity of the blood, solving the problem of the tendency of these patients to develop "sludged blood," which interferes with circulation. That reduction in blood viscosity would also be a service to the elderly, whose circulation often needs all the help it can get.

The emphasis on marine oil obviously invites the consumption of more oily fish, or a supplement of these oils. The principle is applicable to those who want to use every protection against heart and blood vessel disease, but it also could be applied for those who are already following diets low in cholesterol and animal fat. Your doctor, if the diet was prescribed by him, should be consulted. Those on the Pritikin diet must wrestle with the inventor's prejudice against fats and oils, which should have been modified when the more liberal American Heart Association diet was found as satisfactory.

EPA has applications other than prevention of cardiovascular disease. Early animal research hints that it may protect against kidney disease, too, though that application in human beings is years away. It may be beneficial in systemic lupus erythematosus, arthritis, and certainly in early multiple sclerosis.

For those who, reading this chapter, have decided to raise their intake of EPA and DHA by more frequent consumption of oily fish, choices are somewhat limited in this country. They include salmon, mackerel, sardines, and anchovies. If you choose to supplement your diet with these marine fats in capsule form, such supplements are already available in the health food stores. There you will also find pyridoxine (vitamin B_6) concentrates in potencies ranging from 5 or 10 mg. up to 100 mg. However, your need for supplements will not stop there, if you raise your intake of EPA and DHA. Such highly unsaturated fats create an increased requirement for antioxidants. That subject is explained in Chapter 5. Read it carefully. Not only do the antioxidants in nutrition protect fats (like marine oils) against "rancidity" in the body, but they retard aging and they are a potent protection against some serious diseases.

The marine lipid concentrates currently available appear in capsules containing 180 mg. of EPA and 120 mg. of DHA. Physicians might for therapeutic purposes prescribe a number of capsules daily. For prevention, the manufacturer's supplementary dose should be your guide.

There is the tale of the little child who asked if there were any vitamins in a doughnut. When his mother said there were none, he responded with the incredulous "You mean it's just for fun?" I'm sure the average wine drinker would subscribe to this description for his favorite beverage; but there appear to be several dividends from regular consumption of modest amounts of *red* wines—advice that is obviously not intended for alcoholics, dry or not. Alcohol has been found to elevate the high-density lipoproteins, and red wine contains phenolic compounds with antiviral effects. One is reminded of Rabelais's remark that there are more old drunkards than old doctors, but strict moderation is the key to these putative benefits, which suggest routine use of perhaps two glasses of a good wine daily. The term "good" doesn't refer to a good year or a palatable wine. The laws that strictly govern the use of various additives in wine have a number of loopholes for foreign imports, making it judicious to select an American wine you find palatable.

Another dietary factor that may prevent a host of unpleasant and sometimes lethal diseases is fiber. I have already called your attention to its neglected importance, as evidenced by the wholesale removal of fiber from the processed foods preferred by Americans. I mention fiber here because it tends to slow the absorption of fats and cholesterol from the diet, making it easier for the body efficiently to metabolize these factors. This is an important consideration for the elderly, in whose blood the fats and cholesterol of a meal linger many hours longer than they do in the young. Because I have already rejected cholesterol and fat as *the* explanations for hardening of the arteries and heart disease, I take a dim view of those who have described fiber as *the* sovereign protection against these disorders. It may help, as any normalization of the body's metabolism may; and there is cogent evidence that a few extra grams of fiber daily may aid you toward a healthier and younger old age. The subject deserves close inspection, which I give it in Chapter 10.

In a country of hasty breakfasts, lunches snatched on the run, and dinners that are often the only decent meal of the day, the final suggestion for protecting the arteries would probably require legislation to force adoption. However, the timing of meals is as important as their composition, and it is unphysiological to eat three meals a day. That schedule is a concession to bus and train schedules and the work calendar, but fails signally to meet the needs of the body. Smaller and more frequent meals stabilize blood glucose levels, make weight control easier, and dampen the effect of dietary cholesterol on blood levels. The principle is sound, the effect easy to understand. The body can cope with protein, fat, and carbohydrate in large amounts, because it must, but the less efficient organism pays a price. Smaller meals make smaller demands on the mechanisms of absorption and utilization. For hypoglycemics and sufferers of tinnitus and Ménière's syndrome, this meal pattern—perhaps five small rather than three large meals daily—is mandatory. For the rest of us, it is preferable.

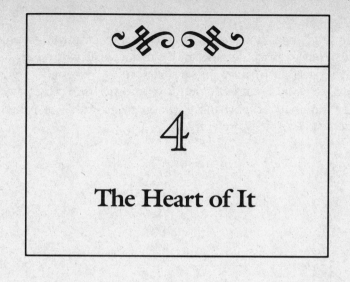

4

The Heart of It

DOCTOR TO ELDERLY PATIENT: "Stop complaining. I can't make you younger."

PATIENT TO IMPATIENT DOCTOR: "I'm only asking you to make sure I grow older!"

Medicine has, if anything, encouraged the public's belief that growing old causes disease. This was the message physicians gave us when they said: "Normal blood pressure is your age plus one hundred." It means that you "normally" grow sicker every year. So it is that the increase in heart and blood vessel symptoms, year by year, has been accepted as inescapable, average, and therefore normal. In an experiment which, like so many valuable studies in the field of nutrition, has been given unwholesome neglect, University of Alabama medical researchers showed that there is the possibility of diminishing, rather than increasing, the symptoms we suffer as we grow older. Moreover, they specifically pointed out "the potential of accomplishing this goal by simple dietary means."

For this study, they examined the interrelationship between vitamin E intake and cardiovascular findings. In the members of the group who consumed insufficient vitamin E, they did find the "normal" relationship between clinical symptoms and age. Among these subjects were some who, for the next year, increased their intake of the vitamin. Only for these was there a decrease in the cardiovascular findings. Specifically, the practitioners reported: "the clinical picture of the group improved approximately 30 percent . . . the average fifty-year-old had become more like a forty-year-old within twelve months."

Question to my reader: what is your vitamin E intake? If you eat white bread, processed cereals, and regard the use of wheat germ as a practice of health nuts, your intake of vitamin E may be low enough to threaten that advancing years will bring growing troubles with your heart and circulatory systems. It is relevant that consuming increasing amounts of polyunsaturated fats, cherished by the low-cholesterol enthusiasts, can create a deficiency in vitamin E.* For the vitamin to exert its full protective effects, it must be accompanied by selenium. It is interesting that veterinarians for years have treated angina in animals with a combination of the two nutrients, but except for a group of physicians in Mexico, clinical use of this simple, harmless nutritional formula in the United States is rare, though the Mexican trial showed a significant reduction of angina symptoms.

Many years ago, the noted surgeon Dr. Alton Ochsner used vitamin E and calcium as a preoperative treatment. His aim was to reduce the incidence of clots and blood vessel inflammation, common complications after some types of surgery. He reported that this simple precaution sharply cut down on postoperative thrombophlebitis.** Prevention of death from a second heart attack was the objective of Dr. James P. Isaacs of Johns Hopkins, who treated twenty-five patients, veterans of severe heart attacks, for ten years, using daily supplements of vitamin E, vitamin C, zinc, manganese, copper, and estrogen and thyroid hormones in small doses. Statistically, one would expect thirteen of twenty-five heart disease patients

---

*Such fats can also interfere with the favorable effects of the marine oils, described in Chapter 3.

**Patients taking anticoagulant drugs should not take vitamin E, for the effects may be additive and thereby excessive.

to die within a ten-year period. Two died. The study has been expanded to a much larger group, and we are awaiting this report.

From what you have read, you have learned that vitamin E is an anticlotting factor. My good friend Dr. Wilfred Shute, who has used the vitamin to treat some thirty thousand heart patients, has shown that it helps to dissolve existing blood clots. There is ample evidence that it improves the transportation of oxygen by the red blood cells, and simultaneously makes the heart a more efficient pump by reducing its need for oxygen. Many of the public, at least those sophisticated in nutrition, have learned that topical application of vitamin E minimizes scar tissue formation after burns and other lesions. That same action is exerted by vitamin E after an infarct, preventing excessive scarring that would, of course, diminish the efficiency of the heart muscle. Finally, vitamin E dilates the capillaries, thereby improving circulation. I have seen demonstrations of a temperature rise in the legs of patients with compromised circulation who were given vitamin E. Dr. Richard Passwater notes that veterinarians capitalize upon the reduced need for oxygen afforded by vitamin E, and give it to race horses regularly.

When the action of vitamin E in preventing deaths from heart disease is examined, one discovers that it exactly parallels the effects of the marine lipids. It reduces the adhesiveness of the blood platelets, which makes for a reduced tendency to blood clotting, and the blood becomes less "sticky"—viscosity is reduced. It also slightly reduces the number of platelets, but like the marine oils, it doesn't carry this to the point where hemorrhaging tendencies are caused. It is interesting that garlic also reduces excessive adhesiveness of the platelets, indicating that the folklore concerning this popular seasoning has a basis in fact.

There is clear evidence that vitamin E acts to protect the cell membranes against carcinogenic chemicals and compounds that can cause the cells to grow abnormally, creating the type of damage which may start the process of atherosclerosis. In the cardiovascular system, vitamin E is an extraordinarily useful unit of the nutrition family, for it benefits both the heart and the blood vessels. To what extent it does this was the question addressed by Dr. Passwater. Acting on the theory that what nutrition helps or cures, it may prevent, he investigated a large group of vitamin E supplement users for frequency and severity of heart attacks. He found a significant correlation: the more vitamin E they took, and the longer they had taken it, the fewer heart attacks they had. Critics might well point to uncontrolled variables in this study, citing the possibility (or probability) that people who take vitamin supplements may be people who don't smoke, but that consideration doesn't erase the correlation Dr. Passwater found among duration of use, potency of the supplement used, and infrequency of heart attacks.

I have given you a *very* small sample of the scientific findings that emphasize the importance of adequate intake of vitamin E in achieving a healthy old age. When you read Chapter 5, on the antioxidants, you will encounter evidence that the aging process itself may be slowed by these factors, including, of course, vitamin E.

If you react to this discussion as many of my university students have, you will be wondering why your family doctor has never suggested the use of a vitamin E supplement. Aside from the point made earlier—that medical schools which don't teach nutrition graduate physicians who minimize its importance—there is also the cultural lag in medicine, epitomized in an ancient admonition: "Be not the first to lay the old aside, nor the last to adopt the new." It reflects a philosophy that creates a constipation of new ideas. When I lectured at the Albert Einstein School of Medicine, a student remarked: "If nutrition were important, they would make it a required rather than an optional course."

A good example of the medical logjam in nutrition is found in a case history involving vitamin E therapy, told by Dr. Wilfred Shute, whose brother had hospitalized a patient with thrombophlebitis, which is inflammation of blood vessels, complicated by a clot. The first day, beginning vitamin E treatment, he put a notice on a bulletin board, calling his fellow physicians' attention to their opportunity to observe the woman's response to vitamin E therapy. He updated the notice, reporting her progress, on the second day. On the fifth day, when the woman was discharged from the hospital after an accelerated recovery that would not have been attained with drug treatment, he posted his last bulletin, recording the therapeutic victory. But in those five days, not one physician had accepted his invitation to observe the results of the therapy.

There have been negative reports on vitamin E, but, as one

medical nutritionist remarked, if those reports had been *favorable*, they would have been rejected as anecdotal and therefore untrustworthy. There *are* a few instances where the vitamin must be administered with caution. These include individuals with underactive thyroids, those with rheumatic heart disease, and those—particularly the elderly—with hypertension. Raising blood pressure is not a characteristic of the vitamin, but a response stemming from an idiosyncrasy of the user. In all these instances, the vitamin *is* administered under medical supervision, usually starting with very small and gradually rising doses.

The rest of us will often profit significantly by use of a vitamin E supplement, which is a remark based on an actual study of vitamin E levels in a random sample of American adults, the majority of whom had inadequate blood levels of the nutrient. (The research was conducted at Tulane University.) However, you don't start by buying the first brand suggested at your drug or health food store—a remark that invites explanation.

Vitamin E appears in a number of forms, all designated by the term *tocopherol* prefixed with a Greek letter. Those of interest to us are the alpha, beta, gamma, and delta tocopherols. The alpha form is the most active in intracellular chemistry, but the least active as an antioxidant. (See Chapter 5.) The delta, gamma, and beta forms are the efficient antioxidants, in descending order. These you will find labeled "mixed tocopherols" or "vitamin E complex." Potency will be stated in units of alpha tocopherol alone, and the content of the other tocopherols will not be stated, though I should like that custom to be adopted. At any rate, the form of vitamin E containing only alpha tocopherol should not be your choice.

Through my fifties and sixties, I was taking 400 units, as mixed tocopherols. In my seventies, I have doubled that, with consideration of lessened efficiency of absorption and utilization. Unless, though, you are minded to wear my shoes and eyeglasses, you should not predicate your intake on my choices, for each of us is biochemically unique. In the twenties and thirties, one might start with 200 units daily, raising that to 400 from the forties through the sixties. Increases after that will be influenced by the impacts of the aging process, which, if this book accomplishes its objectives, will be minimal.

The fact that selenium and vitamin E depend on each other has inspired some manufacturers to market combinations of the two. Avoid these, for they are invariably overpriced, as compared with the cost of using each nutrient separately. Guidance in purchase and use of selenium is discussed in Chapter 5. Likewise, avoid the water-soluble or emulsified forms of vitamin E. They're often alpha tocopherol alone, and usually overpriced. You can improve absorption, which is the intent of these emulsified forms, by using lecithin with the fat-soluable vitamins A, D, E, and K. Lecithin, discussed in Chapter 5, is another in the group of antioxidants that may help to retard aging and to dampen one of the processes that may lead to cancer. It shares with vitamin E and marine fish oils the properties of lowering blood cholesterol and—what is possibly more important, as you now know—raising the level of the protective high-density lipoproteins. The frequent reference to this type of protection should not lead you astray. No more than low blood cholesterol guarantees freedom from atherosclerosis and heart attacks do high-density lipoproteins confer absolute safety. To cite just one neglected factor, stress to which a person can not accommodate is very efficient, no matter what the diet, in raising blood cholesterol. This has been shown in students at examination time and in accountants at tax time. When the stress affects an individual with a compulsive type of personality (the so-called type A), blood cholesterol rises and clotting time decreases. The nutrients we have been discussing are valuable in limiting these adverse responses to stress, but given that type of personality, one needs behavioral conditioning, which can be accomplished and can be effective. Books on the subject are beginning to appear, and some psychiatrists are already addressing the problem in appropriate patients. An excellent text on the subject and a good investment for those who are compulsive, try to do two things at once, and live and work under constant deadlines, is *TQR—The Quieting Reflex,* by Dr. Charles Stroedel, published by Putnams.*

These are people who have never had a heart attack but nevertheless develop angina, ordinarily the cry of a damaged heart that is being overtaxed. For want of an explanation, medicine called

---

*Behavioral psychology isn't your only resource, if your personality creates or magnifies stresses to the point of threatening your cardiovascular system. For many people, biofeedback and Transcendental Meditation are effective antidotes. Many holistic medical centers teach these techniques.

this "aberrant angina," which explained nothing; but an explanation was found when surgeons, viewing the naked heart during a bypass operation, witnessed a heart attack in the absence of the clot (coronary thrombosis) classically supposed to be *the* cause. A spasm swept through the coronary arteries that supply blood to nourish the heart muscle, drastically reducing the flow of blood. Magnesium deficiency has been linked with the tendency to spasm, and abnormally low levels of the metal have been in the hearts of those perishing with sudden heart attacks. Backing up these observations is the inverse ratio between the hardness of water and the incidence of heart attacks: that is, where the water is hard, the heart attack rate tends to be low. In one community, switching from a soft-water to a hard-water supply was followed by a 48 percent reduction in heart attacks. There is also calcium in most hard water, and between the two nutrients there is an interplay, calcium being vital to the contraction of the heart, and magnesium to the reversal of the contraction, allowing the heart to rest. It may seem contradictory to you that physicians are using calcium blockers to help troubled hearts, but what you have read indicates that the procedure would reduce the contractility of that organ, so that it is subject to less demand. You will note that no one has suggested the use of a magnesium blocker, which would probably cause arrythmias.

If you live in a soft-water area, as evidenced by the lack of need for water conditioners and by the easy lathering of soap, protection of your magnesium intake is obviously sane. Foods rich in magnesium are almonds, barley (not pearled), lima beans, Brazil nuts, cashew nuts, corn, whole wheat products, hazelnuts, oatmeal, peanuts, peas (fresh), pecans, brown rice, soy flour, and walnuts. Distilled water will of course supply no magnesium, nor anything else but water, and should be avoided, but a good mineral water for drinking, reconstituting frozen fruit juices, and other beverages purposes is a good investment. Query the spring water supplier, for some of these products come straight from the tap rather than a spring. Magnesium levels need not and usually are not high; the amount of water we need is large enough to make it a valuable source of minerals.

Probably the best-utilized form of magnesium supplement is magnesium orotate. This is only 8 percent magnesium, yielding about 33 mg. of magnesium in a 500-mg. tablet, but the metal is efficiently absorbed by the body from this source. If the orotate type is used, at least 100 mg. of magnesium—the content of three 500 mg. tablets—would be required. If other types of magnesium concentrates are employed, such as dolomite, the need may rise to 400 mg. daily.

Raising the body's magnesium level isn't an exercise in simple arithmetic of more intake equals more storage. It can take years to elevate low magnesium levels, and it may require dropping some amenities, including smoking, the convivial cocktail, and the use of coffee and tea. So reports Dr. Gary Gordon, who probably knows more about mineral metabolism than most of us. For him, it took five years to raise body levels of the metal to a normal amount. I myself, consuming an excellent diet rich in magnesium sources for many decades, discovered that I was *90 percent* short of normal levels of the metal. This, not at all incidentally, was not established by hair analysis. For many good technical reasons, hair values alone cannot be used as an index of surplus or deficiency of essential nutrients. It is reliable alone only in appraising body loads of heavy metals, such as lead, cadmium, and arsenic.

I mention this because I am concerned by some health professionals who place too much weight on hair analyses alone, and I am even more concerned when such analyses are used by nutrition counselors, some of them practicing in health food stores, who on the basis of hair analyses urge their clients to purchase large quantities of vitamin, mineral, or protein supplements. No competent medical nutritionist would endorse that advice. He would know that a high zinc level in hair may represent excessive excretion, which has actually caused a zinc deficiency; that a low level of magnesium in the hair could reflect conservation by the body, with resulting normal levels in tissue and blood. Hair analysis is a unit in a necessary series of tests, and cannot stand alone.

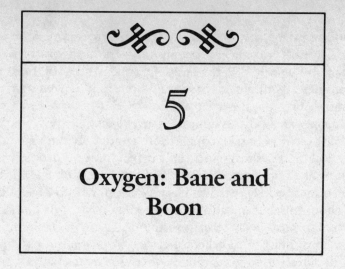

5

Oxygen: Bane and Boon

Oxygen supports the flame of life. It is linked with the treatment of life-threatening diseases, as its use in the emergency room constantly reminds us. Some of the symptoms we call "senility" bespeak a brain not receiving enough oxygen. When blood circulation is compromised and insufficient oxygen is reaching the tissues, gangrene is but one of our worries. How, then, can oxygen become bane rather than boom? You might think about that question the next time you see a steel bridge being painted for the specific purpose of keeping oxygen from attacking the beams.

To understand how oxygen turns into an aging agent rather than a support of life, let's return to a subject in Chapter 3. We were discussing polyunsaturated fats, which in high intake can prematurely age the skin. Such fats are highly unstable, which is a scientific way of describing what the public would call "likely to become rancid." When such "rancidity" occurs in the body, a chain of events follows that may open the door to premature aging and to cancer. When a polyunsaturated fat breaks down in the body, it becomes a source of what the chemist calls "free radicals." These are highly reactive substances which, chemically speaking, are restless because they are lacking the normal number of electrons. Seeking to repair that lack, the free radicals will, among other undesirable characteristics, react with available oxygen molecules, and out of that union will come a highly active form of oxygen, peroxide. The peroxides are toxic and capable of damaging and, indeed, destroying cells. If you wish to translate that into its effect on longevity, these reactions are responsible for shortening the life span by 10 percent in animals fed a high intake of polyunsaturated fats. The remedy for this is not avoidance of such fats, for we need a modest intake of them. The remedy is found in the antioxidants, such as vitamin E, for this nutrient sacrifices itself to reduce free-radical reactions, thereby blocking the oxidation that can turn fats into harmful peroxides. Since the vitamin is sacrificed to give us this protection, the supply must be renewed regularly, which means every day. The chemist would say that the body regularly requires a supply of free-radical scavengers. You might think of vitamin E and other antioxidants as little Pac Men, pursuing and gobbling the free radicals before they can work their mischief.

There is a long list of such natural antioxidants with which—if you want to stay young—you should become acquainted. Intercepting the reactions that create activated oxygen, though, is only one of their functions. Consider, for example, some of the characteristics of another member of this family, glutathione. It is an antioxidant and a deactivator of the free radicals. It is also an anticancer agent, frequently a characteristic of antioxidants. It plays an important role in the immune system. It is used as an aid in the treatment of allergies, cataracts, diabetes, and hypoglycemia, and as an anti-inflamatory agent in arthritis. It helps you to utilize iron and the sulfur-containing amino (protein) acids, such as cystine and cysteine. Given by mouth, it is more effective than superoxide dismutase, an antioxidant better known to the public. Glutathione accelerates respiration in the brain. It helps to protect against the toxic effects of cigarette smoke and those of alcohol.

There are so many antioxidants in nutrition that one wouldn't suppose that peroxides would survive long enough to make mischief. The list includes the bioflavonoids, and vitamins A, C, and E, B_1, pantothenic acid, PABA, lecithin, B_2, beta carotene, inositol, choline, and cysteine. Sometimes the nutrient isn't an antioxidant but participates in reactions that create one. Niacinamide is one example. Even cholesterol may act as an antioxidant, which explains the drop in serum cholesterol when some of these nutrients are given. The body wisdom depresses the cholesterol when other, less willful antioxidants are provided.

In autopsies on the very aged, a pigment has been found, long called "senile pigmentation." A similar pigment, though, appears in the bodies of animals deprived of vitamin E. Although they are not chemically identical, the pigments share one characteristic: their appearance isn't owed to aging, but to deficiency in the antioxidant, meaning vitamin E.

The havoc created by activated oxygen logically suggests that lowering the supply of oxygen should be helpful. The body, though, doesn't work that way. High oxygen levels quench the formation of the peroxides; low levels stimulate peroxide formation, but lack the quenching effect. In either case, a generous supply of the antioxidants is obviously indicated. This means that treatment with hyperbaric oxygen, which has been used for the senile, among other indications, should be accompanied by generous amounts of the nutritional antioxidants. It isn't, for this is another of the many areas where medicine is guilty of a cultural lag. The same could be said of alcoholics; for heavy drinkers, by a clearly understood chemistry, are heavy producers of free radicals, and need all the protection they can get against hyperactive oxygen. Free radical production is also high in those exposed to automobile exhausts and in cigarette smokers as well as alcoholics, and people subject to these toxic influences particularly need high intake of vitamin C, B_1, and the sulfur-containing amino acid, cysteine.

The allergic profit by the antioxidants, too. They are important in offsetting the side effects of autoimmune reactions and asthma attacks, where free radicals, a type of oxygen called "singlet," and peroxides are released inappropriately.

The brain is not only vulnerable to the attack of free radicals, but obviously puts the antioxidants to other good uses, for doses of them have been reported to raise the IQ and improve mental function in the elderly with reduced supplies of oxygen to the brain. The high polyunsaturated fat content of brain tissue makes it vulnerable to free radicals, and this is apparently anticipated by the body, for that tissue contains one hundred times as much vitamin C, an excellent antioxidant, as other organs of the body. This may be part of the reason for the usefulness of vitamin C levels as a predictor of survival, even more than smoking, obesity, or alcoholism as a negative factor. You can apply this observation to your search for a diet and supplement regimen that will help you to stay younger. It translates into simple arithmetic: those with higher levels of vitamin C in the blood, statistically speaking, can be expected to live longer. The real problem isn't in achieving that; it is the dose needed, which varies tremendously from person to person. Dr. Linus Pauling told me that the range of requirement goes from 250 mg. to 2,500 mg. daily. Though this outrages those who want to feed people a little more vitamin C than you need to prevent scurvy, which is a ridiculous philosophy, that range is far less than that encountered in animals, which may have requirements varying by a factor of thirty.

The immune system, which tends to decline in effectiveness as the years accumulate, is a target for free radicals, too. It is believed that their targets particularly are the hypothalamus (the part of the brain where the autonomic controls are housed) and the pituitary gland. Free radicals also strike directly at the programming of the cells, where the "blueprints" are stored, in the DNA. The creation of one small error in those blueprints could, for example, upset limitations on cell division and growth, which would be a pathway to cancer. So it is that superoxide dismutase and other antioxidants are found helpful in protecting DNA.

Since this discussion has emphasized the tendency of fats unprotected by antioxidants to form free radicals, it should be obvious that those who are well larded with fat—the obese—must be at risk of an onslaught of free-radical formation, and so it proves, this possibly being the reason for their marked susceptibility to a number of diseases. The same mechanism is operative when we are X-rayed, diagnostically or therapeutically. Many of the side effects of radiation derive from its potency in creating free radicals. This explains the improved tolerance to radiation in the well nourished, though, unfortunately, those who are so treated are, if anything, more likely to be malnourished.

The chemists who enter the field of nutrition tend to make peroxides, free radicals, and antioxidants the central theme of their approach to the field of nutrition. In fact, before I wrote these lines, I listened to a tape of an hour lecture on nutrition by a chemist, indicting free radicals as the primary causes of all degenerative diseases. Listening to such one-note players in the nutrition orchestra, one could easily decide, depending on which savant one trusts, that antioxidants, peas and beans, and whole wheat will wipe out senescence and everything from cancer to atherosclerosis and heart disease. On paper or orally delivered, it sounds convincing, but theoretical chemistry can stub its toe when applied to the complexities of man. To illustrate what I am saying, consider that I offer a chemist a compound that is readily metabolized by the body, ultimately broken down into water and carbon dioxide. Surely it must be harmless? If the chemist is unwary and assures me that it is, what will he say when I tell him the compound is alcohol?

At the same time, I don't want to diminish the importance of antioxidants in our nutrition. They do help in building resistance to disease by protecting the immune system; they do slow the processes that could otherwise accelerate aging; they do protect us to a great extent against some of the inimical influences we can't entirely avoid, such as radiation (some of which comes from space). I have profited by raising my intake of antioxidants, and most people do, but they aren't panaceas, and in the responses to this chemistry there are individual differences, as there are in all human and, indeed, all animal responses.

There are synthetic antioxidants, widely used in industry. You have seen "BHA" and "BHT" listed on the labels of food products and described as preservatives. I recently read a eulogy of BHT for human use as an antioxidant, and found it difficult to believe that anyone would choose so suspect a synthetic chemical in lieu of effective and harmless nutrients. BHT was found, years ago, to depress the levels of three liver enzymes, and feeding it to animals in pregnancy was followed by the birth of 15 percent of the young without eyes. Japan has banned its use in the food supply. The British restrict its use to salad oils, and allow only very small quantities. We swallow this material in hundreds of foods, and taking it by the spoonful seems a gratuitous journey into the unknown. Otherwise, why would the World Health Organization have condemned the use of BHT in baby foods, and why has the FDA recently announced that questions about the safety of this compound have been raised, and that it is under reexamination? I suggest that you bypass the spoonful doses of BHT and restrict yourself to the nutritional antioxidants, which convey benefits without question marks.

And now let's learn something about a factor of the vitamin B complex, para-aminobenzoic acid, with some fascinating actions in preventing and, indeed, in treating some of the disabilities we blame on time itself. This was the first antioxidant I used personally. Dividends accrued.

PABA:
A Nutrient That Slows Aging

In Boston, many years ago, practiced an endocrinologist who was years ahead of his time. Though medicine ignored it and still does, he was aware of the interplay between vitamins and hormones, so intimate and complex that a deficiency of one might show up only as a lack of the other. So it was that in his correspondence with me, there was language like "mixed vitamin-hormone imbalance." In contrast to this display of understanding of endocrine-nutrition interrelationships is the remark made to me by the chief of endocrinology at a major New York hospital, who said, "I could tell you all that I know about nutrition in five minutes!" and looked astonished when I suggested that he had just disqualified himself for the practice of glandular medicine.

The Boston physician, Dr. Benjamin Sieve, acting on a hunch he never explained, decided to treat female infertility with a nutrient, para-aminobenzoic acid. This, which we shorthand as PABA, is a factor of the vitamin B complex, not officially considered a vitamin because the body manufactures it and thus, theoretically, requires no external supply of it. The assumption that each of us synthesizes enough PABA to meet our needs, though, is highly iffy. If that were so, we should not see, as we often do, remarkable responses to supplements of PABA. Such responses appeared in Dr. Sieve's trial of the nutrient in the treatment of twenty-two infertile women, all of whom had tried unsuccessfully to become pregnant, for a period of five years or more. Given a few hundred milligrams of PABA daily, twelve of the twenty-two had successful pregnancies within two years. Which invites the question: what has this to do with aging? It is pertinent if you remember my earlier description of premature senility in children (progeria) as being caused by pituitary deficiency. When PABA stimulates fertility and when it retards or reverses graying of the hair, which it sometimes does, the long odds are that this reflects stimulation of the pituitary gland.

PABA interacts with both estrogen and cortisone. The helping hand it gives to the female hormone has been useful to women who have low estrogen levels. Female hormone activity in women differs by a factor of more than five, and those at the low end of the spectrum may age prematurely and go into early menopause. PABA is also synergistic with cortisone (that is, they help each other to work more effectively), thereby aiding the body in meeting stress without overburdening the adrenal glands. That interplay could be, but rarely is, capitalized upon by physicians prescribing cortisone, though the use of PABA would permit lower dosage of the hormone, which is always inviting when you are using a drug with an unbelievable list of side reactions.

In the late 1950s, my interest in PABA was keen, for I'd already seen it recolor gray hair, stimulate fertility (there are babies, born to previously infertile parents, for whom I am a nutritional godfather), and slow down the aging process. Then there came from Rumania the first of a series of papers on the results of administering PABA to the aged. The story was essentially that of slowing or reversing the impact of aging. The physician performing this research was with the staff of an old-age home, and I obtained permission for one of my medical consultants to visit the home and observe the rejuvenating process. He was fascinated by what he saw, to the point where he returned to the Rumanian clinic three times in a period of some ten years. When my consultant, Dr. Herman Goodman, first visited the clinic, he found Dr. Anna Aslan treating a group of elderly patients, many of them too feeble to leave their wheelchairs or beds. In the ten-year period, he was able to appraise the response of that group for the decade, and found that the treatment had turned the clock back for many of the aged patients, some of them now able to function, even to the point of performing small chores in the nursing home. Cognition had improved, wrinkling was less apparent, gray hair had recolored, and energy levels were higher.

American medicine paid little attention to Dr. Goodman's reports, and less, if anything, to Dr. Aslan's papers. One physician did try the experiment of giving PABA to life prisoners in a New York State prison, and found that the prison diet, low in PABA, rather than the rigors of imprisonment, is responsible for the premature gray hair of many convicts, for he secured a distinct darkening of the hair in a number of his subjects.

Actually, the Rumanian physician was not using PABA in the usual tablet form in which it appears in our health food stores. She was injecting a form of procaine, which you know under its trade name as Novocaine, the local anesthetic your dentist uses when he patches the teeth you have insulted with the average American diet. That local anesthetic, though, is a combination of PABA with a solvent, and it later devolved that both the solvent and the PABA contributed to the physiological benefits.

PABA, as its full name—para-aminobenzoic acid—indicates, is an acidic vitamin, and some people do not tolerate acids well. (This is also true for niacin and ascorbic acid.) If this is a problem, we use the potassium salt of PABA, which has the virtue of not being an acid; it is also more soluble (dissolves more readily), making for better absorption. However, potassium-PABA is, for no discernible reason, obtainable only with a prescription, for physicians use it to treat arthritis and allied painful disorders. I have been known to jest that the orthodox physician who prescribes it for arthritics doesn't realize that PABA is a vitamin, and will assure you that there is no nutrient that helps arthritis.

There are other dividends from raising the body's supply of PABA. One of these comes from minimizing cross-linkage of proteins. To understand this phenomenon, which contributes to wrinkling as you grow older, think of protein (amino) acids as parallel strings of beads, side by side, with few connections between the beads on one string and those on its neighbors. When cross-connections are established in an abnormal degree, which is cross-linkage, you develop reduced elasticity of the skin, which you've been blaming on old age. Many other nutrients help PABA to minimize cross-linkage, including cysteine (supplied by eggs), vitamin A, B_1, B_2, pantothenic acid, B_6, vitamin C, zinc, and selenium. The inimical effects of excessive exposure of your skin to sunlight are minimized by beta carotene, from carrots and green vegetables, and by PABA. Carotene is available, concentrated, as a supplement.

As we age, we are reminded by our physicians that the immune system weakens, and told to be sure to report for shots of flu vaccine. That weakening of the immune system, which is discussed in detail in Chapter 8, can be offset by vitamins C, E, and A and the minerals zinc and selenium. Note that many of the nutrients that minimize cross-linkage and premature aging of the skin also help you to resist both infection and cancer.

One of the problems faced by our astronauts was premature death of red blood cells. These cells have a limited life, normally, and are replaced by the body, but in space, the life span became abnormally short. The NASA nutritionists apparently forgot their homework, for PABA, inositol, and choline help to protect the red blood cells. In space, the astronauts were exposed to larger amounts of radiation than we earthbound citizens are, and that irradiation, some of it probably cosmic in origin, has an adverse effect on cell membranes. Within our cells are "garbage disposal" units called lysosomes. When the cell membranes are penetrated by irradiation, the acid enzymes within them, intended to dispose of cellular debris and intended to operate only within the confines of the lysosomes, spill into and begin to digest the structure of the cell itself. The factors that increase the longevity of red blood cells exposed to radiation also help to protect the lysosome membranes. All this adds up to a potent weapon against premature death of cells, which translates into an anti-aging force of considerable potency. Not incidentally, this action of nutrients can be usefully employed to help patients who must undergo therapeutic irradiation, for some of the side effects of such treatment involve the mechanisms we have just discussed. The membrane-protecting effect is also partially responsible for the helpfulness of PABA in allergic asthma, for allergy often induces excessive permeability and weakening of cell membranes.

I have experimented personally with PABA, both as such and as the potassium salt, as well as with injections of procaine. Dr. Anna Aslan is insistent that her procaine formula for injection differs only slightly from the Novocaine formula, but that the difference is significant, and her preparation (GH3) thereby more effective. I have not been able to confirm that, and for years have used potassium-PABA, 500 mg. daily. I did use Novocaine injections, but found self-administration difficult. Let me note that Dr. Robert Atkins, whose expertise in medical nutrition I accept, tells me that he has been using the GH3 injections personally, finding them more effective than Novocaine by injection or PABA by mouth. These conflicting reports should not be allowed to deprive you of the long list of benefits of PABA, in one form or another, for its anti-aging and other effects. In addition to the fact that it occasionally darkens gray hair, it intensifies the normal pigmentation of the nipples and the mucous membranes of the mouth, vagina, and anus; it eradicates areas of vitiligo (depigmentation of the skin) for some of its victims; it reestablishes the menstrual cycle in amenorrhea (stopped menstruals); it occasionally stimulates the libido, benefits some asthmatic patients, increases appetite, and induces a feeling of well-being. In addition to other actions, PABA has been shown to be an effective detoxicant for arsenic and many other types of poisoning. I should note that its effect in stimulating the response to the female hormone estrogen would obviously not be desirable for women with disorders triggered or worsened by that hormone, including the prolonged menstrual, marked premenstrual symptoms, cystic mastitis, uterine fibroid tumors, and breast or uterine cancer. But for the opposite group, low in estrogen, PABA may help to preserve the characteristics of youth that so often tend to slip away with the menopause.

PABA is available in 100-mg. tablets in the health food stores and is used in supplementary intake in doses of 500 mg. daily. The prescription form, the potassium salt of PABA, is available only in 500-mg. tablets or capsules.

VITAMIN C (ASCORBIC ACID):
Antioxidant, Anti-Aging, Life-Prolonging

Many years ago, when I was director of education for a laboratory headed by Dr. Casimir Funk, originator of the term *vitamin,* we formulated the first multiple vitamin-mineral supplement to be introduced to the medical profession. As I look back over the decades to that formula, I am struck by the modest amount of vitamin C it provided. This, though, was in accordance with the thinking of that era, which, unfortunately, is still characteristic of the minds of those who regard as generous any amount of a vitamin adequate to prevent a deficiency disease. In the case of vitamin C, that would be scurvy, and the amount needed to prevent it, believe it or not, is just 10 mg. daily. However, the functions of vitamins go beyond keeping your foot out of the grave, and vitamin C is an excellent example of that.

In the aging process, an important factor is the degeneration of collagen, the "glue" that binds our cells together. It is caused by the factors we have been discussing: peroxides, free radicals, radiation, cross-linking, and, always in the background, stress. The amount of vitamin C needed to prevent scurvy may be grossly inadequate to protect collagen against degradation. Keeping collagen molecules young and in good repair is an important role of vitamin C in slowing the aging process. You can't stay younger than your years if, literally, you are coming "unglued."

This nutritional antioxidant is obviously important to our bodies, which contain so many components sensitive to oxygen, while we live in an environment rich in the gas. Animals have met the challenge better than we, for most of them retain the ability to manufacture the vitamin internally and are not dependent on the elusive supply in food. Somewhere in the long history of evolution, man lost that function, and today we are in the precarious position of depending on food for supplies of this essential factor. I say "precarious position" because vitamin C, being an antioxidant, has a penchant for combining with oxygen, which turns it into dehydroascorbic acid, which not only fails to perform the functions of vitamin C, but also has undesirable effects. As an example, injecting dehydroascorbic acid into animals has caused diabetes.

Particularly striking is the ability of animals to raise their vitamin C production to astronomical heights when under stress. This is obviously a protective mechanism, and again, we lack it. Research indicates that the adrenal glands, which produce some fifty hormones we need to resist stress, are enormously concentrated in vitamin C, but lose much of it when the hormone output is raised to meet stress. These pressures being forces in accelerating aging, we now have a second role for the vitamin, one that again indicates that the small amounts needed to prevent scurvy are far below the amounts for long life and good health. As the Roman dramatist Plautus said, who but a god goes unwounded all the way?

While appetite may fail, and idiosyncrasies of taste may likewise militate against optimal diet for the aged, the fact is that ascorbic acid requirements *increase* as the years accumulate. In an examination of twenty-five supposedly normal elderly individuals, only two of the group, aged sixty to eighty-three, had normal ascorbic acid retention. This means that the large majority retained large percentages of a big dose of vitamin C, a phenomenon which indicates that the wisdom of the body recognizes the need and refuses to part with the nutrient. At any rate, higher vitamin C requirements and lower levels in the elderly body have been reported by numerous investigators. In a fascinating project with a large group of the elderly, aged sixty to ninety years, a physician studied the effect of vitamin C on the production of adrenal hormones. Low body levels of the vitamin and low output of the hormone went together, but a single injection of 500 mg. of ascorbic acid sharply increased the hormone level, and that effect was maintained in subsequent ascorbic acid treatment. The essential point in this should be obvious: if the aged over the years had been generously supplied with the vitamin, their adrenal function would have been maintained. Stress being the negative factor it is, and ascorbic acid being so directly important to the function of the adrenal glands, which are the source of our antistress hormones, this says that those generously supplied with ascorbic acid should retain into old age the resilience of youth in meeting the "slings and arrows" of life.

Another dividend from generous intake of vitamin C is the support it gives the immune system. This was clearly evidenced in the cancer research of Linus Pauling and his collaborator, Dr. Ewan Cameron. Failure to realize that the responses of their cancer patients to vitamin C therapy represented the benefits of stimulation of the immune system was the egregious mistake made by the Mayo Clinic doctors when they attempted to repeat the Pauling-Cameron research. They ignored Pauling's warning that chemotherapy depresses the immune system, that vitamin C is helpful in cancer because it stimulates that system, and that its usefulness is therefore compromised if the patients have previously been treated with chemotherapy. In effect, he was telling the Mayo group that patients subjected to previous chemotherapy must be excluded from the clinical trial of vitamin C in cancer. The Mayo Clinic ignored the warning, and their results were predictable: no benefits from vitamin C. This unforgivable stupidity hid from the public and the professions the fact that the vitamin is useful in treating cancer, and that, in turn, promises dividends from generous intake of ascorbic acid as a factor in prevention. (While the Mayo Clinic never pleaded guilty to the error, they announced that they would repeat the experiment, this time eliminating patients with prior chemotherapy. It is over a year, and we are still waiting for a report.)

While massive doses of vitamin C are deliberately given in a single dose or multiples for some conditions, the best way to capitalize on the anti-aging, immune-system-stimulating effects of ascorbic acid is to keep the blood levels routinely high. This either calls for more frequent, smaller doses, or for the use of a time-release form of the vitamin. However, the usual time-release formulation is made with resin or wax—the theory being that the body will dissolve the little pellets at varying intervals. The theory is fine, but the practice not very effective. In the case of vitamin C, however, one company has solved the problem by using a formulation in which the crystals are embedded in a matrix from which the body must free them. This is more successful than the wax or resin types. This product, made by the Schiff Company, is available only in a 1,500|mg. potency. Since we estimate the range of requirement to be between 250 and 2,500 mg. daily, this formulation will be useful only to those with the high requirement. The 2,500 mg. ceiling isn't sacred, and 3,000 mg. could be used. For those with lower needs, ordinary ascorbic acid tablets are, of course, adequate, though they should be taken at intervals to achieve the total dose, rather than all at once.

There is a test for blood levels of vitamin C, but I have already discounted the value of such an appraisal. There is also a test for tissue concentration of the vitamin. This is accomplished by injecting a dye (indophenol) in the tongue and gauging the tissue vitamin C level by the length of time it takes for the vitamin to decolorize the dye. This gives a picture of the vitamin at work in the body, rather than the largely meaningless blood level. Another test measures the vitamin C content of the white blood cells. This, too, is a functional test, because the white cells are part of the immune system and are less active if their vitamin C content is low. Your doctor should be familiar with this appraisal, which measures the ascorbic acid content of what is known as the buffy layer of the cell.

Although it may seem to you that I have told you more about vitamin C than you thought you wanted to know, this discussion actually is distinguished more by its omissions than by its statements. You'll find much worth knowing in *The Healing Factor* by Irwin Stone, published by Grosset and Dunlap. It offers information on vitamin C in relation to the common cold, viral and bacterial infection, cancer, the heart and vascular system, strokes, arthritis and rheumatism, aging, allergies and asthma and hayfever, mental disease, and numerous other disorders.

Other than laboratory tests, the ultimate appraisal of your own individual need for vitamin C comes from your subjective reactions. How you feel and how you function may not impress medical doctors as a means of determining optimal vitamin C requirement, but can be for you the most sensitive and reliable test.

Since ascorbic acid *is* an acid, there are those with sensitive digestive tracts who will not tolerate it well. If sodium intake is not a critical factor, such individuals can use sodium ascorbate. If this is not desirable because it is tantamount to using salt, there are numerous other ascorbic acid compounds, including calcium ascorbate and magnesium ascorbate. Individual differences frequently appear in reactions to vitamin C in any form. A common intolerance is revealed when vitamin C, usually in large doses, causes loosening of the stool or outright diarrhea. This is usually dose-related, which means that the problem can be solved by identifying the dose which causes the reaction and maintaining intake a little below that level.

A few words should be said about side reactions imputed to high vitamin C intake. Most of these allegations come from propagandists for the drug and processed food industries, masquerading as objective scientists. They have warned the public about kidney stones, gout, sterility, and infertility, all supposed to result from high-level intake of the vitamin. A recent communication to *Lancet,* a respected medical journal, reports that the vitamin offers no threat to individuals in good health, and that includes kidney function. The allegation concerning fertility must amuse female schizophrenics who have been helped with 60 *grams* (60,000 mg.) of the vitamin daily and have remained fertile despite ten years of such therapy. There is one side reaction that *is* accurately described. It is called a "rebound reaction." With large intake of the vitamin, the body elevates its output of the enzymes that break down vitamin C. If you stop the high doses abruptly, the enzyme levels don't fall, at least for a few days, and their activity can temporarily render a low dose totally inadequate. The answer to that is obvious. Don't stop abruptly. In fact, unless you have a good reason and your health is good, don't stop.

SUPEROXIDE DISMUTASE

Another of the body's defenses against activated oxygen is the enzyme superoxide dismutase (SOD). It is a highly efficient member of that family, but not in the tablet form in which it has been purveyed to the public. Doses of superoxide dismutase taken by mouth are not well absorbed, and significant blood levels are not achieved. Given by injection, the action of SOD is much more effective; still more so if it is provided in the form in which it is actually used in the body. There it is joined by copper and zinc. For some years, veterinarians have employed this type of SOD in animal disorders, one frequent application being the enlarged prostate, similar to that in man, to which some breeds of dogs are subject. Injections of this veterinarian material, known as Orgotein, have spared these animals from the indignity of prostatectomy and orchiectomy (castration). Ironically, the veterinarian use of copper-zinc SOD evoked no curiosity in the genitourinary specialists, who have no effective nonsurgical treatment for the condition in man. Nor did its successful use for arthritis in race horses.

Superoxide dismutase, which is concentrated from cow's liver, has also been successfully employed in the treatment of early human cataract. In this application, the SOD is dissolved in DMSO, a solvent, and used as eyedrops. This should not invite self-medication. Too strong a solution of DMSO can harm the eyes, and there is a hazard in diluting the solvent: if it is done improperly it generates heat and can explode. I will send information about the formula to doctors upon request.

The limited yield in blood levels of SOD doesn't mean that supplements of the enzyme, for those who want youth to last longer, aren't worthwhile. However, those who are allergic to milk must be cautious, because of the bovine source of the enzyme. Dosage is specified on the product label.

LECITHIN

Not only an antioxidant but a potent regulator of cholesterol, lecithin can play a double role in slowing aging. Lecithin, like a soap, is a very powerful emulsifying agent. This explains its use by the food industry in dispersing fats more uniformly in their products. In the body, it has a similar function, tending to emulsify (dissolve and carry away) cholesterol deposits. In fact, an ideal ratio has been proposed: in the blood, there should be slightly more lecithin than cholesterol, something in the order of 1.2 to 1. When this is achieved, the blood cholesterol can be high, and yet show no tendency to produce fatty deposits.

It has been pointed out, primarily by those who try to belittle modern nutrition, that lecithin is synthesized in the body and that external sources are therefore both unnecessary and unproductive. One would never guess that there have been repeated studies of the benefits of lecithin supplements, showing a strong regulatory action on blood cholesterol levels. Not only are there dividends from a dietary supply of lecithin, but there are rewards from increasing the intake of the factors from which the body manufactures it. These are methionine, which is an essential amino (protein) acid, choline, and inositol, which are directly involved in synthesis of the factor. Other nutrients play a background role in lecithin synthesis in the body, these including vitamin B_6, magnesium, and polyunsaturated fats.

The integrity of the body's cell membranes may be dependent on lecithin, among other factors. Formation of prostaglandins is another of its functions. It helps to keep red blood cells apart, important in maintaining oxygen supplies to the tissues. Foods like milk and soybeans are rich in lecithin, but the supply in eggs is not useful, for that is a different type of lecithin. If you decide to supplement your diet with the granules, you will need one or two tablespoons daily. Three times that amount has been used to help patients with angina, but those with weight problems will find an obstacle in the 100-plus calories in each tablespoonful of the granules.

The lecithin granules you will find in the health food store are adequate for the antioxidant and emulsifying roles of lecithin. However, you may notice on the shelves another type, usually labeled "high-phosphatidyl choline lecithin." This formulation is used not for antioxidant and emulsifying actions, but for its role in promoting the synthesis in the brain of a neurotransmitter, acetyl-choline. Raising brain levels of that transmitter has been found helpful to short-term memory in both the aged and the senile, as well as those suffering from a side reaction to Thorazine tranquilizers, called tardive dyskinesia.

Those allergic to soy, not an infrequent sensitivity, may find commercial lecithin supplements, which are made from that bean, a source of gastric symptoms. Until recently, this barred the use of lecithin for such individuals, but lecithin concentrated from animal brain tissue has appeared on the market, made by the Dews Company, Mineral Wells, Texas.

SELENIUM:
A Powerful Antioxidant

It isn't unusual in the history of nutrition to find a palpable error monotonously repeated as fact. The name for vitamin E reflects that, for it is not the "reproductive factor," yet the name *tocopherol,* which means "childbearing," reflects that misunderstanding so long perpetuated that changing the name would not dispel the mythical linkage of the nutrient with an aphrodisiac effect. Selenium has also been subjected to the same order of misunderstanding. For decades, it was mistakenly considered to be nutritionally useless and, indeed, hazardous, both highly toxic and carcinogenic. Despite research showing, if anything, that selenium is a potent anticarcinogenic agent, as recently as late 1982, a reputable nutrition organization warned the public that use of selenium supplements is irrational, unrewarding, and highly dangerous.

Those abreast of more recent information are aware that this mineral is an extremely powerful antioxidant and, ironically, a potent protection against cancer. In fact, there are some of us who are aware that ineffective chemotherapy for lung cancer became therapeutic when selenium was added to the protocol. At any rate, epidemiological evidence, certainly available to the viewers with alarm, clearly indicates that adequate selenium intake may be woman's best protection against breast cancer. This awareness derives from the experience of Japanese women, who are highly resistant to breast cancer when living in their native country, but become as susceptible as Caucasian women when they move to and live in Hawaii for about ten years. The change to our type of diet appears to be the only reasonable explanation for their increased incidence of breast cancer, and the primary difference is in the high fish intake, rich in selenium, in the Japanese diet, as compared with the yield from typical American menus. The difference is considerable; a Japanese woman cuts her selenium intake by about 50 percent, in the process.

Anticancer effects are proverbial for antioxidants. In the case of selenium, there is a double-barreled action, for this mineral interlocks with vitamin E, which is itself, as you now know, a good antioxidant. The vitamin is much less effective when adequate selenium does not accompany it. The chemistry is not yet understood, but the implications are plain: keeping a careful eye on your selenium intake is likely to be rewarding. Epidemiological studies within the United States clearly show an inverse relationship between soil selenium levels and both cancer and heart attack rates. Moreover, in animals there is a type of heart disease that can be produced by means of selenium deficiency, resulting in the heart muscle's losing its structural integrity. The disease occurs in man in some other areas of the world, but as yet is very rare in this country, perhaps because at least some selenium is provided, even by the atrocious American choices in foods. One case was reported in 1982 in a New York child. At any rate, selenium is a constituent of an anti-aging enzyme, glutathione peroxidase, and an essential nutrient, not to be neglected.

There is a parallel between selenium and chromium. While the body can utilize very small amounts of these nutrients in their mineral form—as selenium and as chromium, or salts of these—utilization is best when they are available in the "bound" form. This explains my preference for selenium supplements such as concentrated brewer's yeast, where the mineral is bound with protein, in preference to sodium selenite or other salts. Most health food stores carry the yeast-derived form of selenium, and the usual potency is 50 mcg. (one microgram is one-thousandth of a milligram). There should be no problem with this small potency, since the difference between the U.S. and Japanese selenium intakes is far greater. We average 300 hundred mcg. daily; the Japanese, about 500 mcg. By weight, the difference is small, but the effects can be weighty. Perhaps you will appreciate that if you consider the text of a letter written by a chemist to a chemical journal, in which he finds fault with many of the experiments with the carcinogenic effects of various chemicals, for, he says, no attention is paid to the basic diet of the animals, and "balanced" diets of differing composition can differ significantly in their selenium content, thereby lowering or raising the resistance of the animals to cancer.

ZINC:
The Missing Antioxidant

In the early 1940s, an FDA agent found fault with a multiple mineral supplement on the grounds that 5 mg. of zinc constituted a toxic dose, and, in any case, zinc supplementing was supererogative, for deficiency in the metal was impossible with any diet that sustained life. I displayed for the inspector a bottle of an antacid, which in the recommended dose contained twice the amount of zinc in the supplement. That ended the argument, but didn't end zinc deficiency in America.

Though zinc is involved in perhaps a hundred different enzyme processes in the body, American intake of this antioxidant is so low that a single day of fasting may produce recognizable symptoms of deficiency in the nails, months later. If you wish a dramatic exhibition of the importance of this long-neglected antioxidant metal, attend a dance of young teenagers, and note that the thirteen-year-old boy is almost invariably shorter than his female counterpart. Zinc is so heavily used in the maturation of the male genitals that growth is sacrificed to this purpose.

Zinc acts as an antidote for the copper overload that may accrue from copper-piped soft drinking water. It is also an antidote for cadmium, a metal believed to contribute to the toll of hypertension. Dry prostate tissue (human) contains 50 percent zinc, explaining the beneficial effects of zinc treatment for the benign enlargement of the prostate in elderly men. Zinc is supplied by whole grains and meat. In supplements, it is usually offered as the gluconate, though other forms of chelated zinc are also marketed. The gluconate tends to be less costly than other forms, and is well utilized, particularly if vitamin B_6 is taken with it. Supplementary doses of zinc shouldn't go overboard, for the antagonism to copper can be a source of mischief, when copper levels aren't excessive, and deficiency in copper is a menace, too. To obtain the 15 to 30 mg. of zinc recommended as a supplementary intake, one must carefully read the labels, for the gross weight of the tablet isn't the gross weight of zinc. Thus one must watch for the phrase "yielding —— mg. of zinc" to distinguish between tablet weight and yield of the metal.

PANTOTHENIC ACID *(Calcium Pantothenate, Pantothenol)*

Since I have had the pleasure of appearing on the scientific platform with Dr. Roger Williams, who discovered and synthesized pantothenic acid, I can give you firsthand information concerning his attitude toward the "official" requirement listed in the RDA for this nutrient. The recommended dietary allowance is between 4 and 7 mg. daily, whereas Dr. Williams finds that many individuals profit by an intake of 25 to 50 mg. daily.

Among its many roles in the body, this antioxidant vitamin has the task of converting choline (an antioxidant) into acetylcholine, which is a neurotransmitter important to memory, among other functions. Even more critical is the role of pantothenic acid in supporting the function of the adrenal glands. Since these are an essential component of our stress-resisting mechanisms, pantothenic acid intake can make the difference between unsuccessful and effective resistance to stress. Stress being the real factor behind elevated blood pressure, blood cholesterol, heart attacks, and other plagues of modern man, any help the body can get should not be limited by the scribbling of the authorities who assume that all Americans are biochemically identical, face identical stress, and thereby have identical requirements for nutrients, including pantothenic acid.

What with the roles of the adrenal system in supporting the immune functions, in regulating blood sugar, and in meeting the emotional and mental pressures faced by modern man, a daily supplement of pantothenic acid makes biological sense. Sometimes called vitamin B_5, pantothenate is found in whole grains, legumes, and animal proteins.

High doses of pantothenic acid have been helpful in rheumatoid arthritis, and in intercepting the ulcer-creating impact of stress on the stomach.

VITAMIN B_6 *(Pyridoxine)*

The role of vitamin B_6 in possible prevention of atherosclerosis has already been discussed in Chapter 3. That, though, is only one of many actions of the vitamin important in retaining youth and mitigating the tolls concomitant with aging.

B_6 sometimes increases the flow of tears, allowing contact lenses to be worn by those whose eyes were formerly too dry. Coupled with exercise, taking vitamin B_6 increases the output of human growth hormone, an action promising help for hypoglycemics, for this hormone raises blood sugar. The effect theoretically, though not yet tested, could be important to children dwarfed for lack of the hormone. The vitamin has value in preventing motion sickness, the nausea of pregnancy, and postoperative nausea. Given with zinc and manganese, it is a specific remedy for pyroluria, which is the cause of a type of schizophrenia. It has also been found helpful in drying the excessive oiliness of the skin which contributes to some outbreaks of acne. In the aging and aged, vitamin B_6 has a particular usefulness, since it helps the body to conserve protein, thereby minimizing the loss of tissue mass so characteristic of some aged people. As an antioxidant, pyridoxine has proved valuable in arthritis, for some of the degenerative changes in that disease are owed to free radicals, for which it is a scavenger. The vitamin is also used to treat carpal tunnel syndrome, which in the opinion of some researchers is actually a vitamin-B_6-deficiency disease. Pyridoxine increases the absorption of zinc, explaining why the two nutrients are often used together, as they are in prostate enlargement. Women find vitamin B_6 a good friend, for it acts as a natural diuretic for the retention of fluid in the premenstrual week. In my own research, I have found pyridoxine helpful for muscle tone and a stimulant to energy. All told, it is an important nutritional weapon for those who treasure good health and a productive middle and old age. The more so, because it is intimately involved in the production of a neurotransmitter that, among other actions, is needed to prevent depression. For the adult, 10 mg. of pyridoxine daily is the recommended minimum. There are those with a significantly greater requirement, among them sufferers with an adverse reaction to monosodium glutamate, who suffer headaches, flushes, and gastric distress after eating Chinese foods or any of the numerous food products in which the flavor-enhancing effect of monosodium glutamate is employed. The "Chinese restaurant syndrome," the title given to the intolerance of the seasoning, is regarded as a specific symptom of vitamin B_6 deficiency or dependency, the latter being the term for a requirement far higher than that of most people.

Autistic children have been significantly benefited by supplements of pyridoxine. The elderly, who frequently can use all the help they can get in the utilization of fat and protein, also profit by augmented intake of the vitamin. Finally, there are epileptics and others, a minority of the population, to be sure, who have a metabolic impediment in the utilization of pyridoxine. For them, we use pyridoxal-5-phosphate, a form of the vitamin which enables them to bypass the fault in the metabolic pathway.

While the authorities set the B_6 requirement even lower than the one they assign to pantothenic acid (about 2 mg.), an optimal intake for many individuals may be between 10 and 25 mg. daily. If you reread the discussion of atherosclerosis in Chapter 3, you will realize that the high intake of methionine in the American diet is a threat to the arteries if insufficient vitamin B_6 accompanies it. With this consideration, and the importance of the vitamin to the function of the brain and nervous system, a generous intake is an insurance policy for old age.

VITAMIN A

You have already learned that an intake of vitamin A beyond the RDA is associated with greater life expectancy. If you've been reading the newspapers, you know that vitamin A (and C) is now considered an important weapon against cancer, by the same authorities who a few years ago assured us that only quacks invoke diet as a protection against malignancy. However, if you have encountered those verities, you probably have read that vitamin A is a two-edged weapon, because "it's toxic." Let me clear the propaganda away, first by telling you that toxicity isn't a property of a substance; it's the property of a *dose*. *Anything* is toxic—blondes, water, oxygen, if you're exposed to enough of it. The vitamin A "toxicity" story is just that: a story capitalizing upon the public concept of the term, promulgated by those who regard vitamin supplements and natural foods as a threat to orthodox medicine, Jell-O, and cornflakes.

Only if you have read the bibliography provided by the FDA do you realize that the adverse reports on vitamin A have been taken out of context. One case "proving" the toxicity of vitamin A involved a four-month-old-baby, dosed by the mother with several hundred thousand units of the vitamin daily. Another was that of a four-year-old, given some 500,000 units of the vitamin daily. The cases were blared from the media, and no one noticed that the children had been given about one hundred times the RDA. Accordingly, when I testified on the issue, before a congressional committee considering the FDA's desire to "protect" the public by requiring prescriptions for vitamins, I demonstrated that multiplying the average intake of coffee, salt, or quinine water by a factor of one hundred would also reach the toxic—indeed, the lethal—level; and logically suggested that coffee, salt, quinine water should be available only on prescriptions, too.

This story I have told you because I have encountered many intelligent health professionals, including physicians, who have been taken in by this propaganda tour de force. I am not proposing that you dose yourself with gargantuan amounts of vitamin A, but I am strongly suggesting that the evidence is compelling that 5,000 units of the vitamin daily is *not* the ideal intake for the considerable percentage of Americans whose nutritional requirements exceed the statistical guesses of the Washington computers. Several points need to be emphasized:

1. There are, in the hundreds of years of use of cod liver oil and, more recently, vitamin A concentrates, only two case histories I've been able to find where doses below 50,000 units daily elicited symptoms of toxicity.

2. The toxicity of vitamin A is reversible, quite simply, by lowering the dose. In fact, in German physicians' management of cancer, frequently million-unit doses of vitamin A are used, and if toxic symptoms appear, the dose is simply lowered.

3. Conversely, injections of 100,000 units of vitamin A have been used successfully to treat hearing disorders caused by otosclerosis. Likewise, quarter-million-unit doses, administered daily for a week, have been used successfully to abort colds. Similar dosage has been employed to treat premenstrual syndrome.

With the importance of the vitamin as an antioxidant, and very specifically, its joint role with beta carotene (vegetable vitamin A) in resistance to cancer, it is a pity that this campaign of denigration of the vitamin has been permitted to obscure the facts. Those include studies at the University of Alabama, where a physician who is an authority in the field of nutrition has correlated intake of vitamin A with health levels, and finds that requirements range from 10,000 to 33,000 units daily, with distinct health advantages for those who meet their needs adequately.

Oddly enough, our manufacturing processes, in concentrating vitamin A from fish liver oils, may have placed us in the position of throwing the baby out with the bathwater. I have been suspicious of that for many years, and have long suggested that it is better to use cod liver oil than the vitamin A and D concentrates marketed as such, or as part of multiple supplements. Understand that I had no quarrel with supplements of vitamins A and D, for I am fully aware that the housebound elderly, among other groups, receiving no sunshine, may develop the weakness of the skeleton that makes them so subject to fractures. However, I had an uneasy feeling that the other components of fish liver oil, other than the vitamins, were more important than we realized. That, a pure hunch, has been confirmed in studies of Greenland Eskimos, living on their high-fish diets, as compared with us and with Eskimos who have migrated to Canada and to the Canadian (modern) diet. Mortality rates from heart attacks among the primitives on high intake of oily fish is 5 percent. In the "modernized" primitives, eating our foods, the rate leaps to *50 percent*. This effect has been traced to a fatty acid in fish oil called eicosapentaenoic acid. Its effects include lowering elevated blood cholesterol and triglycerides, decreasing the adhesiveness of blood platelets (which minimizes the type of clots that may initiate atherosclerosis), and making the blood less viscous (more slippery), thereby improving circulation. Because cod liver oil is so rich in vitamins A and D, there is a limit on the amounts nutritionists would recommend, and for that reason, marine lipid (fat) concentrates, largely free of the vitamins, are now being marketed. My hunch about the baby and the bathwater was prophetic.

All this explains the presence in health food stores of marine lipid concentrates, offered as a supplement to the diet. Questions remain to be answered: for instance, the dramatic improvements in blood chemistry have been achieved by doses of 5 grams of eicosapentanoic acid daily for a few months. We do not know if lower doses for a longer period would have the same effect. If that so devolves, it will avoid the need for swallowing a massive dose of eicosapentanoic acid capsules, for the present potency is less than 200 mg. of the acid per capsule, which is a fifth of a gram, requiring some twenty-five capsules daily to reach the 5-gram level of intake. If you will forgive another hunch, I believe that a much lower intake for a much longer period will prove equally rewarding. In collaboration with the American Institute of Stress, I am now investigating that. The marine liquid concentrates create a fascinating opportunity to offset the physiological impact of stress, for that is really the factor behind elevated cholesterol, atherosclerosis, heart attacks, and many other diseases. That is why merely lowering blood cholesterol is an exercise in futility: it attacks the symptom, not the cause. If marine lipid concentrates will let us block even part of our stress reactions, they will save countless lives.

Until all the facts are in, it would appear to be a good investment to take cod liver oil in the manufacturer's recommended dose. If there is a family history of atherosclerosis and cardiac deaths, or if your physician finds that your blood chemistry is in the risk range, the marine liquid concentrates deserve discussion with your practitioner.

BETA CAROTENE

The importance of being earnest about vegetables in your diet is emphasized by the discovery that high intake of vegetable vitamin A, which is beta carotene, is a key to resistance to a number of types of cancer. Before credit is fully given to this natural antioxidant, there are some points of confusion that must be resolved, for there is some evidence that the anticancer effect may also be attributed to chlorophyll, which is the plant equivalent of hemoglobin. Since you consume both in the same foods, the point would seem academic, but the distinction is important to nutritionists. The next question mark concerns the body's conversion of beta carotene into vitamin A, which is an accomplishment denied to diabetics. This means that those with diabetes can't rely on vegetables for their vitamin A, but must allow animals to perform the conversion, as cows do, thereby providing preformed vitamin A in milk. However, while overdoses of vitamin A can be toxic, overdoses of carotene—even though each molecule creates two molecules of vitamin A—are not. The only penalty for excessive intake of beta carotene is a yellow tint to the skin. One would expect, considering the vitamin A yield from the vegetable precursor, that swigging too much carrot juice would ultimately create too much vitamin A, but this is not so. There is also a mystery concerning the invisible ceiling the body puts on the vitamin A and related compounds the body forms from carotene. This appears to be genetically fixed, which means that there would be an automatic ceiling on anticancer benefits from the vegetable form of the vitamin.

None of this should make you forget that the body doesn't convert all beta carotene into vitamin A. It has uses for the vegetable form, unaltered.

If you are a vegetable hater, and if you find vegetable dishes and juices both unenthralling, your next resort is beta carotene capsules. I note a number of brands tastefully tinted with coal-tar dyes. Patronize a manufacturer with more sense. Potencies range from 10,000 to 25,000 units.

INOSITOL

Another of the free-radical scavengers, this vitamin has suffered the indignity of being labeled a "nonvitamin" by the orthodoxy, for the reason (if it can be called that) that the body manages to synthesize it. Since you have read a similar description of PABA, and now know of some of the dividends from an augmented supply, the "nonvitamin" nomenclature should not disturb you. I learned in the 1940s that supplements of inositol were remarkably beneficial for diabetics, and not until this decade was it recognized that the nutrient helps to speed the transmission of nerve impulses, which, in diabetics, is impeded in the disorder called "diabetic neuropathy." Inositol is also a lipotropic factor, which ultimately means that it helps liver function. Like others of the antioxidant family, it helps to stabilize cell membranes, an important contribution to prolonging youth.

The nutrient occurs naturally in whole grain cereals and breads, wheat germ, fruits (canteloupe is a particularly good source), yeast, lima beans, peas, and organ meats. Supplements of inositol are available, frequently combined with choline. Many multiple supplements contain lip-service amounts of these nutrients, obviously added merely to lengthen the label for impressiveness. A meaningful intake for supplementary purposes would be 1,000 mg. of choline and 500 mgs. of inositol. Higher levels are useful in, for instance, coping with excessive estrogenic hormone activity in women with cystic mastitis, dysmenorrhea, premenstrual syndrome, and uterine fibroid tumors. I must add that I am not impressed by claims made for inositol as a remedy for incipient baldness. It is true that falling hair has an abnormally low level of the nutrient, but it is also true, on the basis of my own observations, that the hair growth encouraged by inositol resembles lanugo, a baby hair, which more or less promptly disappears, too. Nonetheless, what with its free radical scavenging, its effects on the nervous system, and its concentration in both the heart and the brain, this nutrient deserves your attention.

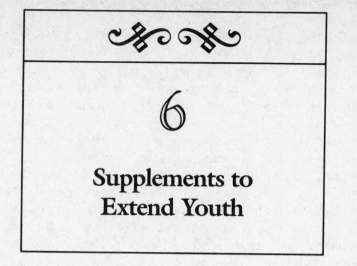

6

Supplements to Extend Youth

In the 1940s, when I introduced the concept of dietary supplements to the public, the reactions ranged from the apathetic to the virulently hostile. This was to be expected, for home economists, whom I described as rarely home and seldom economical, had persuaded the public that good nutrition is guaranteed by appropriate selections from the seven (and now four) food groups. The manufacturers of highly processed foods, with full justification, regarded dietary supplementing as an explicit criticism of their overmilled, overrefined products, and as something akin to condemnation of Mother and apple pie (with twelve teaspoonfuls of sugar per portion). From the ignorant came the argument analogous to that first directed against air travel: if God had intended man to fly, He'd have given us wings. In nutrition, it took shape as: everything man needs from food is provided in it.

This might be true if (a) food had not been changed and (b) we had not changed. I am suggesting that it is imperative that we take advantage of the ability of man's brain to take a detached view of itself and of him. We might begin with the results of a long-ago experiment at Johns Hopkins, where laboratory rats, descendants of thousands of generations of domesticated animals, were compared with wild rats of the same heredity, with both groups subjected to intense stress. The domesticated animals were decimated by the pressures, developing the animal equivalent of "nervous breakdowns" in which they huddled, trembling, refusing to eat. The wild animals fared much better, developing the neurosis one-ninth as frequently. Anatomical comparisons showed significant differences between the domesticated and wild animals. The laboratory rats had smaller brains, smaller stress-resisting glands, and enlarged sex glands, the latter thereby dominating their behavior. When you study the conditions of the experiment, you realize that we provide the domesticated animal with housing, food, water, and mates, while the wild animal faces and is accustomed to the stresses of seeking and sometimes fighting for these necessities. The researcher doesn't acknowledge it, but there is another difference between the two groups: their dietary histories were significantly different, for the wild animal previously selected its own diet, while the researcher decided what the laboratory animal would eat. In the light of the advances in our knowledge of nutrition since the years of that experiment, there is no doubt that the wild animal came to it with a history of better nutrition. Moreover, in such self-selection, the rat is guided by instincts we long ago lost or never had. I am thinking of rats made diabetic, by surgery or medication, which promptly refuse to eat sugar, as compared with the human diabetic who cheats on his diet, though threatened with blindness and the pain of neuropathies for the transgressions. I am also thinking of an incident, years ago, in which a ship laden with whole wheat flour ran aground on the Nova Scotia coast, providing the natives with a free long-term supply of whole wheat flour. During that year, dietary deficiency diseases of two types, which had been common among them, largely disappeared. However, when the cargo was exhausted, the Nova Scotians went back to their white flour and their deficiency disorders. Wild rats would have known better. This, and a thousand anecdotes like it, should disabuse you of a superstition widely held by the public, to the effect that your food cravings are an expression of the wisdom of the body. Do you really think nature built into you a mechanism which expresses a need for a snack of krispy, krackly, devitalized Krunchies?

There is more than food processing as a factor in depletion of our intake of essential nutrients. There is also the impact of a sedentary life, which reduces our gross need for calories but does not lower the nutrient requirements of blood, brain, nevous system, tissues, and organs. Let me present the problem in simple arithmetic. The iron requirement of menstruating women has been set officially at 18 mg. daily. With careful selection of iron-rich foods, one can obtain 6 mg. of the metal with each 1,000 calories from food. This requires a woman to eat 3,000 calories daily. Try that figure for size with any group of women, and you will find, as I have, that given a choice between obesity and anemia, they will unhesitatingly choose anemia. Approach that another way: a diet with less than 1,600 calories per day is on the ragged edge of deficiencies. At 1,200 calories, it requires expert selection of foods to avoid deficiency. Below that, it's impossible. (This is the arithmetic that made us provide the blockaded Berliners with the amounts of food we flew in. The air force would happily have reduced the burden; the nutritionists knew they couldn't.) Yet in the dietary assays my university students submit as part of the course requirements, I find hundreds of diets that are below, and sometimes well below, the 1,600-calorie figure, and among the women, below 1,200.

Surely those who lived during the Revolution, the Civil War, and World Wars I and II considered their times to be uniquely stressful. Where would you rank ours, under the shadow of the atomic bomb, in a world where strife and starvation and unemployment are constant companions? Not to attempt to discuss nutrition versus stress, which would be a book-length essay, consider that the vitamin C content of the adrenal glands is depleted shortly after a major stress, and not regained for months, though the vitamin is essential to the synthesis of the hormones needed for defense of the stress-ridden organism. Translation: we need more generous intake of the vitamin than most diets provide. Interestingly, the animals that do not need dietary supplies of the vitamin, since they can synthesize it, under stress will raise their production to the equivalent of more than 10,000 mg. daily for man. We long ago lost those abilities.

The invention of cooking was a mixed blessing. It breaks down cell walls, making nutrients more easily available. It kills bacteria and other unwelcome fellow travelers. It also destroys or makes nutrients unavailable. Don't discount the losses or the interference with utilization. The prior discussion of the vitamin B_6 losses in food processing didn't stress the point, but this vitamin isn't the only nutrient so affected. As for the influence of heat on the availability of nutrients, consider the babies driven into convulsions and brain damage, with permanent retardation, by the heating of milk formulas, rendering an essential vitamin unavailable to the body, though still present in the milk. The cooking of protein changes it, even mild heat altering it to the point where it can't, for instance, meet the needs of the unborn, the deficit showing in narrowing of the dental arch (which is considered normal because it's average). The effects on behavior thereby go unremarked, though they include "constitutional inadequacy" in women and asocial, violent behavior in men.

Beyond all these considerations, prior to losses of nutrients in cooking, processing, and storage of foods, there is the impact of our agricultural methods. Liming the soil is a standard practice. Unnoticed is the effect of calcium in lowering the magnesium content of the plant. Yet magnesium may be the critical nutrient in protecting us against heart attacks based on spasm of the coronary arteries. Despite the low magnesium value of plants submitted to excessive liming of the soil, the foliage is still lush. Likewise, we are victims of the acid rain from the use of fossil fuels, for this deposits sulfur on the soil. Sulfur and selenium compete for entrance to the plant cells, and a minute amount of selenium will lose the race when the sulfur is dominant, a phenomenon unique to our present culture, and a threat to our immune systems and hearts.

Beyond all this, there is a law of chemistry that gives an advantage to those whose nutrient intake is high. It is the law of mass action. To understand it, consider a tank divided into two watertight compartments by a membrane. We fill both sides with water, but add salt only on one side. By osmosis, the salt will migrate through the membrane until, nature detesting both an imbalance and a vacuum, the salt content of the two compartments is equal. The law of mass action dictates both the transfer and the equalization of the salt levels. It also makes the efficiency of the transfer proportionate to the concentration of the salt—that is, the higher the amount of salt added initially, the quicker the transfer to the other side. For the water, substitute blood. For the salt, a nutrient such as a vitamin or mineral. For the membrane, the wall of a blood vessel or a cell. Now the law operates: the higher the concentration of the nutrient, the faster and more efficient the transfer from blood to tissue or cell. Those who tell you there are no dividends from nutrient intake beyond the recommended daily dietary allowances are obviously trying to repeal a law of physical chemistry. If they are competent, they also know that the recommended daily allowances are *not* intended as yardsticks to measure deficiency or to determine the adequacy of an individual's diet. But a handful of people (thirty-three) in each thousand have their nutrient requirements exactly met by those standards. This isn't academic. It bears importantly on achieving or at least approaching the level of optimal nutrition which is the sine qua non of excellent health and longevity.

Another argument of the skeptics has to do with the roles of vitamins and minerals as components of enzyme systems. The argument has it that the cellular production of enzymes is rate-limited, and you can't accelerate it with higher intake of the nutrients. This is so, but who ever said that we achieve the maximum rate? In Chapter 14 I discuss an enzyme test for adequacy of vitamin-mineral *utilization,* which I described as more meaningful than blood levels of the nutrients. The majority of those so tested prove to be nowhere near their potential for such enzyme production. This isn't academic, for optimal levels of the enzymes are indispensable in retention of health and in retarding aging.

As part of my responsibilities as a public health and nutrition educator, I read thousands of papers and texts each year, culling information important to the public in assuming responsibility for the care of their own bodies. What you are about to read is a sampling of the vast flow of information. It comes from the journals on which your own physician or health care professional depends, and will give you a double view of nutrition: what you do to it, and what it does to you. You'll emerge from the reading with the realization that third-grade nutrition, characteristic of most Americans, produces third-grade health, contributing both to sickness and to shortening of the prime of life, if not of the life span.

The public has learned that a high-fiber diet may protect against hemorrhoids, varicose veins, diverticulosis, diverticulitis, appendicitis, and bowel cancer. Despite the time-honored use of bland diets for many of these disorders, you have also learned that bran supplements are well tolerated by a majority of the sufferers. What you have not learned is coping with the side effects of the high-fiber diet. Increasing dietary fiber may lead to decreased absorption of calcium, magnesium, and iron, as well as lower the blood serum levels of ionized calcium. The high phosphorus content of bran can be an added insult when the diet is already rich in phosphorus, as a result of a high intake of animal protein, which, in the absence of dairy products, will also lower calcium intake. Since high phosphorus intake demands the raising of calcium supplies, the use of bran requires increased intake of a number of minerals, including calcium, magnesium, iron, and possibly zinc. The benefits of a high-fiber diet are too important to sacrifice, but users should be taking a multiple mineral supplement.

Emphasis in diet for reproduction is always directed to the mother's menus and, usually, only after conception has taken place. The factors that affect the germ plasm, though, do not spring magically into action only after impregnation, and affect the father quite as much as the mother. In families with a history of defective babies, vitamin E therapy for the *fathers before conception* materially lowered the number of defective babies in subsequent conceptions and deliveries. Question: how much vitamin E is in your diet? You need it as a potent anti-aging factor, if only to protect reproductive efficiency, and if you are an average American, your supply is inadequate. Those who appear to earn a livelihood by denigrating the values of natural foods and the use of diet supplements have told the public that vegetable oils supply more than adequate amounts of vitamin E. Aside from the point that substantial intake of such polyunsaturated fats may *cause* the atherosclerosis they are supposed to prevent, and contribute to cancer, read the following note from a young man who worked (past tense) for a company marketing such oils:

"I went to our foreman, after hearing your broadcast, and asked him why we remove the vitamin E before we sell our vegetable oils to the public. He told me we sell it to the vitamin industry. When I said I thought that was dishonest and wrong, he fired me."

Some years ago, a researcher at Tulane University decided to test the blood of a randomly selected group of adult Americans for "diene"* content. This is a way of appraising the adequacy of vitamin E intake, since the test appraises "rancidity" in body fats, against which the vitamin is protective. Such "rancidity" is dangerous, accelerating both cancer and aging. He found the test positive in a majority of the group.

Part of the responsibility for protecting yourself against toxic pesticide residues on food is yours. The malign effects of numerous pesticides are increased with deficiency of dietary protein, riboflavin, niacinamide, sulfur-containing amino acids (supplied by eggs), fatty acids, and vitamin C. Vitamin C also protects you against the carcinogenic nitrosamines, formed by the body from the additives used in luncheon meats and frankfurters.

If, after reading the foregoing, you are comforting yourself with the thought that you, like millions of Americans, are eating the "average American diet," heed what the professor of pathology at the University of Chicago Division of Biological Sciences and the Pritzker School of Medicine told the American Heart Association. He had initiated a study of the effects of the average American diet on the coronary vessels of rhesus monkeys, and ran into an astonishing "side effect": the diet proved toxic to the animals, which gained weight poorly, though they were eating more than other animals in the study. They died before the two years of research terminated, and the report of careful gross and microscopic examination of the cadavers did not "help us to understand the reason for this apparently toxic reaction" to the average American diet fed ad lib. As I read this plaintive report, I was reminded of the comment made by a scientist, when radioactive strontium 90 fallout was threatening the Eskimos as a result of its concentration in their usual foods, and the suggestion was made that we encourage them to eat the "average American diet." Said the scientist: "It would fall upon them as a blight." He was talking about *your* food.

"Sugarless" foods, candy, and gum *aren't*. They usually contain a carbohydrate, sorbitol, which is metabolized more slowly than sugar, but has the same role in the body. There is reason to believe that dieters don't realize that sorbitol has the same calorie value as sugar, and that diabetics don't know that, reaching the eyes without normal breakdown in the liver, sorbitol may contribute to the eye disorders considered "complications of diabetes."

---

*Diene is a type of fat resulting from undesirable oxidation of normal fats.

In addition to pesticide residues on food, we must also cope with food additives. We are assured they are safe, though thousands of them have been in use for less than ten years, and the interval between insult and cancer may require twenty. That, though, is but one face of the problem. Additives are tested individually, but we swallow them together, and a distinguished nutritionist has already found interactions among them which increase toxicity or carcinogenicity. At any rate, the next time you read assurance of safety of food additives, write to the author and point out that a dozen food dyes that were pronounced safe in the 1960s are now off the market, as demonstrated troublemakers. Who can give you valid assurances on the current crop? We can, though, tell you that the well-nourished are better equipped to cope with such internal threats.

You're going in for an operation, and you may be slated for a blood transfusion. Statistically, there is a chance, and it's not remote, that you will develop serum hepatitis as a result of the transfusion. That chance diminishes dramatically if you are well supplied with vitamin C. The Japanese demonstrated this with *zero* cases of serum hepatitis in transfused patients pretreated with the vitamin. Question: how's your vitamin C intake?

Your doctor is a low-cholesterol enthusiast, but be of good cheer, for the aberration won't last forever. Nonetheless, you're buying "egg substitute." You're not getting the fine protein of eggs, with the sulfur-containing amino acids which are anti-aging. You're not getting the many vitamins and minerals of eggs, nor the unknown factor that protects against rheumatic fever. But you *are* getting egg white, corn oil, nonfat dry milk, emulsifiers, cellulose, xanthan gums, trisodium and triethyl citrate, artificial color, aluminum sulfate, and iron phosphate—at only twice the cost of real eggs. You can make up the deficit by buying some vitamin E, B_6, B_{12}, trace minerals, and other nutrients alien to substitute eggs but provided by the natural original. What have you been told about the use of supplements? It's unnatural?

The water in your area is hard, and you've invested in a water softener or a still to make distilled water. You're saving on soap, but you've paid a price. Soft water, and none is softer than distilled water, is linked with mineral deficiencies which contribute to heart attacks. Water softeners, in removing the minerals, contribute sodium, no boon to your blood pressure and heart. If you must install a water softener, either leave one line free for drinking water or shift to a mineral-rich spring water or take a mineral supplement.

There's a term you should watch for on the labels of margarine, salad oil, baked products, confections, cereals, and a half-thousand other edibles. It is "partially hydrogenated." This process produces an abnormal amount of a type of fat that disturbs cell membranes, interferes with the production of a vital hormone, and elevates both blood plasma and blood cholesterol levels—the last is ironic when you consider that most margarine buyers are avoiding butter because it is supposed to be dangerously high in cholesterol. American foods contain quantities of these abnormal fats which in Germany would exceed the permitted level by some 2,700 percent!

Your canned tuna, thanks to outmoded packing techniques, may be a contribution to lead poisoning, for the lead in the solder may leach into the contents. Crimped cans, free of solder, are obviously available, for there is at least one brand of tuna fish so packed. Lead poisoning need not be dramatic, revealing itself only in learning difficulties in children or subtle neurological disturbances. The calcium in the diet is a partial antidote, if the lead load is not too great. If your intake of cheese and milk is low, one protection against lead toxicity is missing. In addition, if you want to protect yourself against osteoporosis (weakening of the bones), which cripples and causes disabling pain, particularly in postmenopausal women, that calcium intake will play a double protective role. Question: how much calcium do you obtain?

Contrary to popular belief, flour is bleached not to make it whiter, but to make easier the baking of bubble-gum bread, spongy and filled with air. The bleaching completes the devitalization of the flour in the milling process, destroying vitamin E, carotene, and some 47 percent of the unsaturated fatty acids in the flour. What kind of bread have you been eating?

Another question: in what kind of plastic are you wrapping food? During the Vietnam War, soldiers given transfusions of blood long stored in plastic bags died with "shock lung," which was traced to a leaching of the plasticizer used to make the bag flexible. That plasticizer, a phthalate, is still in use by the food-wrap industry and thereby becomes a threat when it is in contact with foods containing fats. Beating chick heart cells in a culture medium stop beating when they are exposed to minute amounts of the phthalates. To coin a phrase, it's a bum wrap. Don't bother querying the plastic wrap manufacturers, for you'll find their formulas are "trade secrets." If you value your health, in addition to careful selection of food and use of supplements, you'll use aluminum foil, cellophane, or Glad Wrap, which are free of the plasticizer, for foods with a fat content. Generally, the less flexible the plastic, the less objectionable. That isn't the only problem with plastic wrap, though, for in 1973, assays showed a sizable amount of polychlorinated biphenyls (PCBs) in plastic bottles, polystyrene cups, baby bottle liners, bread wrap, and a home-use plastic wrap. The PCBs are highly suspect, adversely affecting the liver, depleting vitamin A reserves and undesirably affecting muscle contraction, nerve activity, and glandular secretions. Carcinogenic effects are still under scrutiny.

There are literally tens of thousands of reports like these you have just read. They don't originate with scare-mongering periodicals, but with reputable and frequently prestigious journals in medicine, biochemistry, enzymology, and nutrition. Were the average person exposed to this information, his selections, from foods to beverages to plastic wraps, would become more cautious. Use of dietary supplements would appear to be no longer an option, but a necessity. That became obvious in Chapter 5 on antioxidants, in which supplements are aimed squarely at an internal chemical problem that promotes cancer and speeds aging.

It has often been suggested that the young man who is courting the young lady should carefully observe her mother, for she is likely to offer a preview of the loved one twenty or thirty years hence. That is the philosophy behind what you are about to read. By examining nutritional deficiencies as they appear in the aged, and their consequences, you can *now* set up what the military calls an "early warning line."

As wrinkles and gray hair aren't necessarily inevitable tolls of aging, but frequently herald it, so are leg cramps. In older people, they often disturb sleep and limit the distance they can walk before pain becomes so great as to be prohibitive. The problem may start with reduced circulation, which can be improved with vitamin E, or it may be caused by a disturbance of muscle metabolism, in correcting which the vitamin has, as demonstrated by its use in angina, been effective. The *Southern Medical Journal* cited the research of two Los Angeles physicians, treating 125 patients with nighttime leg and foot cramps, some of whom had suffered with the painful condition for periods as long as twenty or thirty years. Of the 125 patients, all but two found relief with vitamin E therapy. Of these, 103 had results ranging from "complete" to "nearly complete" control of cramps. Large doses of the vitamin were needed. Smaller "doses" through the preceding years could have prevented the condition. Would you prefer to wait for pain?

If you are a tea drinker, it is worthwhile knowing that the tannic acid in tea can "bind" (make unavailable) about 2 mg. of thiamine (vitamin B_1) if you drink four cups daily. While you're young and have the opportunity for prevention, it would be rewarding to study the effects of mild thiamine deficiency in the aged. They include poor memory, depression, irritability, lack of initiative (which is interesting, because beri-beri means "I cannot" in Singhalese), lack of appetite, insomnia, tendency to tire, inability to concentrate, unsteadiness, and vague abdominal and heart complaints. Tea isn't the only offender. While tea "binds" thiamine, coffee actually destroys the vitamin. So does the use of bicarbonate of soda in cooking vegetables. Would you count it reasonable if I vote in favor of the daily use of a supplement supplying, among other nutrients, a reasonable amount of thiamine? (Don't write to tell me you eat enriched bread, which has thiamine added to it. A few slices are lip service, not a guarantee of thiamine adequacy.)

Folic acid (folate) deficiency can accelerate aging; indeed, it can simulate approaching senility by causing shortcircuits in the nervous system. Patients with this deficiency complained of fatigue, weight loss, insomnia, and severe constipation. Legs were numb and reflexes disturbed. As injections of folate were administered over a period of three months, the subjective symptoms faded, the patients gained weight, and the reflexes returned to normal. This clinical report, which appeared in *Clinical Psychiatry News,* includes an ironic note. All these patients had been under psychiatric care and had been heavily dosed with various medications. A similar report from Scotland describes five elderly patients who had been diagnosed as senile, whose actual problem was folate deficiency. Their nervous systems disorders were so severe that spinal cord degeneration was tentatively diagnosed, but folate treatment resolved the "senile" symptoms, including "severe mental illness" in two of the patients. Question: how many green vegetables are in your diet? How many of them are cooked? It's relevant, for foods boiled for fifteen minutes lose between 60 and 80 percent of their folate. Second question: is it obvious that your daily vitamin supplement should include folate, or do you prefer to wait until it must be given by injection?

A professor of food science at Michigan State University, who authored a discussion of the role of vitamins in the aging process, traced some interesting relationships between diet and aging. He remarked that a higher intake of vitamin C appears to reduce the aches and pains to which older persons are prone, to lower mortality when they are ill, and to increase their longevity. He cited a study in which one of his colleagues measured the average protein and vitamin C intakes of 100 women for a period of almost twenty-five years. Here appeared the direct link between better nutrition and greater longevity, for the women with higher intakes of vitamin C and protein lived longer; in fact, the women who survived tended to raise their intake of vitamin C between 1948 and 1972. Moreover, a striking relationship appeared between nutrient intake and physical health. His report is quite specific: the women who appeared younger than their years consumed less total fat, saturated fat, and fat as a percentage of their total calories, while the women who appeared older had lower intakes of thiamine, vitamin A, and ascorbic acid.

As harsh a measure as it is, the death rate is very often the test of the diet. A study of some 600 people in a California county is a classic in the field. Very accurate measurements were made of the intake of nutrients and of the blood levels of cholesterol, vitamin C, and sugar. Among those whose intake of vitamin A was less than 5,000 international units daily, the death rate in the study period was close to 13 percent. Raising that intake to 7,999 units dropped the death rate to a little less than 7 percent. Among those whose intake of vitamin A was above 8,000 units daily, the death rate was a little over 4 percent, which is less than a third of the rate in the group with the lowest intake of the vitamin. The same results were shown with vitamin C intake. Among those with less than 50 mg. daily, the death rate was about 18 percent. Those who had higher dietary levels of the vitamin had *one-fourth* of that death rate.

In that study, no mention was made of the sources of the nutrients—whether they were derived from food or from concentrates—but there are numerous studies of responses to nutritional concentrates. A pertinent one involved forty elderly patients who were given multiple vitamin concentrates, with a control group given the usual dummy (placebo) tablets. Though the experiment was double-blind, meaning that both patients and physicians were unaware of which group took the vitamins and which the dummy tablets, the physicians could clearly distinguish the vitamin users. At the end of a year of treatment, the physician reporting the study remarked that "there was a striking improvement in the general physical and mental condition" in the vitamin-treated group. He cited as the most dramatic finding in the study the results of stopping the vitamin treatment, for signs of nutritional deficiencies reappeared in many of the previously treated cases. Question: did this superior nutrition extend life, or did it keep life from being gratuitously shortened? The question isn't academic, and you should be acting on its implications *now*.

When you watch the precipitous acceleration of aging in the victim of a stroke, you become sensitively aware that the health of the brain is very much related to extending the prime of life. Since I devoted an entire book to the influence of nutrition on brain function, neurosis, and psychosis, the subject here will receive no more than token examination, obviously. Just consider this: short-term memory has been improved in the aged and in younger, *normal* individuals by increasing the dietary supply of a nutrient used by the brain to make a neurotransmitter, which for the brain is the equivalent of the wires in a computer. Consider the implications of the observation of Dr. Tom Spies, the pellagra specialist: long before the symptoms of pellagra appear, among the earliest evidences of dietary deficiency is loss of a sense of humor. To that you might add Dr. Ruth Harrell's research, which irrefutably proved that the IQ of a severely retarded child could be raised by as much as twenty-five points with a simple multiple vitamin supplement. Conclusion: it is smart to feed your brain optimal nutrition.

Earlier, I acquainted you with the protective effect of adequate magnesium intake on the heart, by way of explaining the lower cardiac death rate in hard water areas. This being the threat it is to the American male at all ages, and to postmenopausal women, let's take a closer look at your magnesium intake. The National Research Council of Canada, listing a variety of causes of magnesium deficiency, also catalogued the illnesses such deficiency might cause. Among their observations was a study of the magnesium levels of the heart tissues of cardiac death, which they found to be 22 percent lower than the level in the heart tissues of those who died from causes other than cardiac disease. Particularly low was the magnesium level in the cases where death came from the classical "heart attack"—lack of circulation to the heart muscle itself. Not only dietary errors, but many other factors can contribute to magnesium deficiency, among them excessive stress, which can increase excretion of the metal.

A medical nutritionist asked me about my own magnesium intake, and I responded with the arrogance of the nutritionist who has eaten a good diet for nearly a half-century, and taken vitamin-mineral supplements as well. He suggested that I not be dogmatic, and ordered tests. I emerged from these chagrined, for my magnesium levels were as much as 90 percent below the acceptable range. I asked the physician what inspired his wariness. He told me that it took him five years to raise his own magnesium levels to normal, and achieving that demanded that he cease smoking, stop the use of caffeine-containing beverages, abjure his social cocktail, and learn how better to handle stress. He added a note important to the reader of a book aimed at extending the prime of life. "Now and then," he said, "I've had the opportunity to check the magnesium levels in the survivors of a family where there have been many deaths from heart disease. The levels are *always* far below what they should be."

Though magnesium is certainly not the only nutrient in short supply in the American diet, deficiency in it is a striking example of those which create health problems we attribute to chance. There are people whose susceptibility to kidney stones subjects them to bouts of crippling pain and the threat of repeated surgery. Some of these are "stone formers." It is a term that makes these people captives of a malign heredity, but new evidence shows clearly that a diet that meets their needs can prevent the disease. One group of patients, about 150, had at least one stone yearly for five years prior to the nutritional treatment. Given magnesium supplements, in the next four and a half to six years, 132 of these patients remained stone-free. Translated into simple arithmetic, this means that an increase in magnesium intake protected almost 90 percent of its patients. Interestingly, the amount and kinds of carbohydrate in the diet also play a role in the problem of kidney stones. The diet high in processed carbohydrates, like white flour, white rice, and sugar, increases the risk of the formation of the calcium type of kidney stone. The risk is increased by Vitamin B_6 deficiency.

Loss of vitamin B_6 (pyridoxine) in such processed carbohydrates and in cooking and freezing foods deprives women of a natural defense against a common symptom in the premenstrual syndrome. In the premenstrual week, many women tend to accumulate fluid as part of their discomfort. Vitamin B_6 has repeatedly been shown to act as a natural diuretic, solving the problem for many women. This doesn't diminish the importance of the nutrient for postmenopausal women. Both sexes, in fact, experience a drop in pyridoxine blood levels after the age of thirty, and the level is cut in half after sixty. Such a loss can play an important part in the wasting of the tissues characteristic of many older people.

What you have read is but a sampling of an enormous literature with which the public will never become acquainted as physicians and nutritionists wedded to the processed food industry create the fallacious impression that all is well with the American diet. The fact is that our culture has made it virtually impossible to achieve optimal nutrition, and the lag in catching up with the truth and helpfully changing your diet will be indefinitely extended if you permit commercially motivated propaganda to substitute for diet. But we have other problems with our nutrition, indigenous to our drug-oriented culture, as you will learn.

Among the nutritional insults we unknowingly inflict on ourselves, there are the negative effects of drugs on our nutrition. This is relevant to the young who would like to stay young, and even more so to the elderly, for the average oldster takes at least thirteen different drugs each year. Among these, barbiturates are offenders, for users have significantly lower levels of blood calcium than nonusers, and barbiturates have been found also to increase the excretion of vitamin C. The same effect on calcium levels comes from anti-inflammation drugs, frequently prescribed to relieve arthritis. Digitalis increases the thiamine requirement, and at least one of the medications for high blood pressure can cause vitamin B_6 deficiency. The antacids destroy thiamine and affect the metabolism of calcium, iron, and phosphorus. The antibiotics interfere with the uptake of vitamin B_{12}, folate, vitamin K, and magnesium. Aspirin does likewise with vitamin C and folate. Cholestyramine, used to lower blood cholesterol, interferes with vitamins A, B_{12}, D, and K. The L-dopa used for Parkinson's disease interferes with vitamin B_6, B_{12}, and folate. Mineral oil—which long ago should have been removed from the market—does a yeoman job in depriving the body of the fat-soluble vitamins, A, D, E, and K. Ironically, vitamin C is an important factor in the body's disposal of many drugs, which means that medications which lower the body's vitamin C levels thereby present a greater risk of toxicity and side reactions.

The relationship between aging and the use of multiple drug prescriptions shows up in the statistics on side effects of medications, for they are seven times as frequent in those over seventy as they are in people, say, between twenty and twenty-nine.

The chances for any of us being hospitalized are in the range of probability. One would suppose that hospital food, fed as it is to the sick, would repair rather than reenforce preexisting dietary deficiencies. Not so: animals fed on hospital scraps have third-grade health, and an assay of hospital meals for copper and zinc, as an example, showed the zinc level one-third below the recommended 15 mg. and copper 50 percent below. Your body needs zinc for many purposes, including healing, and the reserves of the metal in Americans are so scanty that a single day of fasting may cause recognizable evidence of deficiency (as white spots in the nails, months later). You need copper for your blood, certainly also an important consideration for the hospitalized and ill; these, of course, being only a fraction of the uses to which the body puts these metals.

Earlier, I commented on the usefulness of the bioflavonoids in strengthening the smaller blood vessels. You may recall that I remarked that orange juice when strained has lost some 90 percent of its bioflavonoid values, since these tend to be concentrated in the pulp. Yet is not the orange juice served in hospitals, and this under a dietitian's supervision, usually strained? To make that even less forgivable, weakness of the small blood vessels is a problem not only in little strokes but in viral hepatitis, measles, primary atypical pneumonia, mumps, virus A influenza, encephalitis, and other disorders. There are about 3.5 *billion* capillaries in the body, performing the vital task of delivering nutrients and oxygen to the cells and removing wastes. Yet with age, capillary problems become much more frequent. Examination of 189 patients, aged from fifty-three to eighty-eight, revealed 124 of them to be victims of abnormal fragility of the capillaries, particularly in those with high blood pressure. Since hypertension and weakened blood vessels are virtually an invitation to a small stroke, it is instructive to read what happened with victims of such strokes who were treated with bioflavonoids. Ten patients given this nutritional support over a period ranging from twelve to thirty-two months either improved or remained in satisfactory condition, none of them suffering the repeated strokes that are characteristic of the majority of such cases. This note is not gratuitous in a book devoted to retarding aging, for little strokes accelerate senility.

From what I've already written about the diet in heart disease and atherosclerosis, you know that I take a dim view of the extravagant claims made for polyunsatured (vegetable) fats, which in large amounts I regard, with good reasons, as dangerous. With the eulogies of these vegetable oils by manufacturers of margarine and salad oils, you would never learn that frequent use of polyunsaturated oils can make you look old before your time. That is not a theory, but the conclusion reached in an exhaustive study of 1,000 patients who were examined by a plastic surgeon for symptoms of premature aging of the skin. Each patient was carefully graded for crow's feet, frown and worry lines, degree of wrinkling, and such symptoms of skin degeneration as changes in elasticity and color. Seventy-six of the group were women, and the age range was from seventeen to eighty-one. A striking correlation was found between intake of polyunsaturated fats and clinical symptoms of premature aging. In the group who frequently included vegetable oils in their diets, nearly 80 percent showed clinical symptoms of accelerated aging, some of them appearing to be twenty years older than their actual ages. The converse was found in subjects who didn't emphasize the use of vegetable oil in their diets, for 72 percent of them were free of the stigmata of early skin aging. As you will learn, the fallacy of a high intake of vegetable oils derives from their tendency to oxidation (translate as chemical breakdown). The antidotes for that tendency are the antioxidants, so important in resisting aging that I have devoted a separate chapter to that subject.

As you grow older, it is normal for you to require less sleep. In fact, requiring as much or more is sometimes a symptom of insufficient blood supply to the brain. Failure to recognize that normal change in sleeping habits is responsible for much injudicious dosing of the elderly with sleeping pills. If you recall the soporific effects of a glass of hot milk before retiring, you are aware, without realizing it, of the helpfulness of two nutrients in reducing sleep latency—the period between closing your eyes and actually falling asleep. One of these is calcium, and the second is an amino (protein) acid, tryptophane, which in the body is partially converted into a quieting brain neurotransmitter. For some people, this amino acid is given in tablet form, highly concentrated, and has proved markedly helpful to speed the journey into sleep. Interestingly, the same chemistry has been applied to help depression, which is frequent in the elderly. It seems a pity that the insomniac and depressed elderly aren't given this nutritional treatment, which is harmless, rather than the barbiturates, which interfere with calcium metabolism, and the antidepressant drugs with a long list of serious side reactions.

Yesteryear, the test for hydrochloric acid in the stomach was agonizing. Today, a capsule containing a radio transmitter is lowered, attached to a string, into the stomach, and by the wavelength it transmits, the physician can tell whether your hydrochloric acid production is adequate. The point is important to the aging, for with the years come changes in the digestive tract, and frequently among them is a drop in hydrochloric acid secretion, which makes protein digestion less adequate and interferes with absorption of iron and vitamin B_{12}, thereby helping to create anemia. Animal proteins are your only rich sources of the vitamin, but will not be efficient sources if your hydrochloric acid level is low. The physician corrects this by administering a form of the acid, and by injections of vitamin B_{12}, which obviously can't be given by mouth when the problem is poor utilization in the digestive tract. As an alternative to injections, or for added help between visits to the physician, he may recommend sublingual lozenges of the vitamin, to be dissolved under the tongue, where absorption is rapid and efficient.

As the former nutritionist for a major league baseball team, I am aware, as most of the athletes themselves are, of the importance of optimal nutrition to physical conditioning. Often, we use magnesium supplements to improve stamina, and with it, give a concentrate of wheat germ oil, octocosanol, which increases the capacity for muscular effort. But you need not be an athlete to profit by such nutritional safeguards. There is in the scientific literature a report on the effect of magnesium supplements on 100 people complaining of chronic fatigue and low libido. In a double-blind experiment, with one group receiving placebo pills, 87 percent of the magnesium-supplemented group felt stronger. They became more alert, cheerful, animated, and energetic, stating that they rose from sleep with refreshment rather than morning fatigue. All this raises the question repeatedly asked in these chapters: did you have your 400 mg. of magnesium today? And in all the yesterdays? If you don't know, how do you know that your level is adequate, and not threatening you with stress-induced heart attack, kidney stones, or other unwelcome visitors? If you have decided that these questions are not academic, you will read in Chapter 14 about the intelligent use of supplements, to identify the choices that will give you a reasonable chance for better health, a prolonged prime of life, and an aging process that isn't a parade of symptoms and prescriptions.

Middle age has been the focus of nutritional research, too. A British neurologist, back in 1964, arrived at an explanation for "many of the complaints of middle age." He pinned the blame on vitamin B complex deficiency, which he indicted for dysfunctioning of the middle-aged nervous system. Lack of attentiveness, he said, forgetfulness, disorientation, and mood changes are easily blamed on the aging process, but in both the middle aged and the elderly, they can originate with deficiency in this group of vitamins. Responses to vitamin therapy in a few cases may be rapid and dramatic, with symptoms and signs of nervous dysfunction resolving in a few weeks. In the majority, it may take six or twelve months before dimensions of residual disability can be fully assessed. This translates into an echo of an axiom ancient among nutritionists: it is better to prevent than to treat deficiency, for it can reach the point of no return. Even when early enough, nutritional therapy may take a long time to produce responses. In one study, ten of forty elderly patients responded to vitamin dosage in the first three months. In six months, the number rose to twenty-one. At nine months, to thirty. At twelve months, all but one patient had improved, and that one still showed marked symptoms of nutritional deficiency. In fact, contradicting the belief of some nutritionists that high vitamin dosage yields fast dividends in the deficient, at the end of the year some of the patients were still in the process of improving physically and mentally. The milligram of prevention is indeed better than the pound of cure.

When deficiency diseases are mentioned, such as pellagra, beri-beri, or scurvy, the average person thinks in terms of physical symptoms that are flagrant and easily recognizable. Not so. The large majority of us are not deficient enough to arrive at these florid, clear symptoms. We have what I call a "social security" level of nutrient intake. Not enough to live on, not low enough to cause deficiency disease and death. Read a list of the *early* symptoms of a dietary deficiency, in the vitamin B complex:

"There is loss of appetite which is partly responsible for weight loss . . . general muscular weakness, lassitude, irritability, depression, memory loss, headache, and insomnia develop without obvious reasons . . . [plus] nervousness, palpitation, distractability, apprehension, morbid fears, mental confusion, and forgetfulness. . . . Since the entire syndrome often appears without objective cause, a diagnosis of neurasthenia, anxiety state, malingering, or neurosis is usually entertained."

The authority who wrote those lines, a specialist in medical nutrition, emphasized that all this occurs before a deficiency state can be clinically diagnosed. Given those symptoms, without apparent objective cause, and visiting a physician whose medical school did not teach nutrition (a majority of them don't), are you not likely to leave that office with a referral to a psychiatrist or, even worse, a prescription for a mind-bending drug?

Depression in the middle and later years is frequent, and easily and often accurately blamed on financial, social, emotional, and vocational deprivation. Let me trace another cause: you live in a soft-water area, and the piping in your home is copper, a metal that soft water picks up with facility. (Be wary if a dripping faucet leaves a blue ring around the drain.) Elevated copper can cause as many troubles as low intake of essential nutrients. Depression is frequent. So are painful joints, elevated blood pressure, premature baldness, ringing in the ears, facial pigmentation, and insomnia. The medical nutritionist will lower your copper levels with zinc, manganese, or molybdenum, along with vitamin C to flush the metal out. Some people arrive at elevated copper because of deficiencies in the other metals; women do sometimes, through pregnancy or the artificial pregnancy created by the birth control pill. Others are copper accumulators, and need a generous daily supply of zinc and vitamin C throughout their lifetimes, to keep their burden at a safe level. Here you have another of the little things in diet that mold your health destiny.

The considerations that govern your selection of foods are obviously very different from those in the nutritionist's mind as he guides them. Essentially, most people eat what they like, which certainly doesn't guarantee that their diets will meet the challenges with which nutrition must cope: supporting efficient reproduction, normal growth, healthy maturity with needed repair of vital organs, a vigorous old age, and an extended prime of life. To achieve such a guarantee or to come as close to it as possible, I decided more than a half-century ago that in our civilized scheme of things nutritional, there are too many unknowns, and supplementing the diet with concentrates makes sense in the absence of adequate information about our needs and the content of nutrients in our foods. The concentrates, though, are more than an insurance policy, for they offer direct dividends, as you have learned from the discussion of the nutritional antioxidants in Chapter 5.

If you are wondering *what* dietary supplements make sense for *you,* be of good cheer. The basis for the decisions will be found in the last chapter.

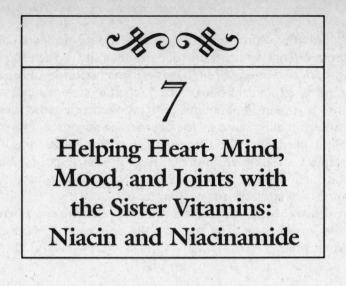

7

Helping Heart, Mind, Mood, and Joints with the Sister Vitamins: Niacin and Niacinamide

"He has lost his spark" is more apt a description of the aging process than one would suppose, for behind reduced supplies of oxygen to aging tissues, in addition to hardening of the arteries, there is a gradual loss of the electrical charge of the red blood cells. In our fifty thousand miles of blood vessels, there are tens of thousands too small to allow passage of the oxygen-bearing red blood cells. To enter and pass through them, the cells not only must bend, but must travel in single file. Order is maintained by the electrical charge that red blood cells carry, making them repel each other, but as the decades pass, the charge weakens, permitting the cells to aggregate. The resulting logjam significantly interferes with circulation and oxygen supply to the tissues. This is, of course, particularly adverse to normal function of the brain and nervous systems.

Seldom mentioned is a vitamin that helps to restore the cellular electrical charge. Usual vitamin supplements don't contain it, and its actions, so far as the knowledge of the public goes, remain one of the ignored dividends of scientific nutrition. That is a preliminary to the story of two forms of the same vitamin: niacin and niacinamide. They were originally called "nicotinic acid" and "nicotinamide." Nutritionists, though, thought the names would persuade the public that cigarettes would provide these factors; hence the change in nomenclature.

Behind niacin and niacinamide is a fascinating history of research with direct application to helping you to stay healthier and younger, both physically and mentally, for an adequate intake of these sister vitamins can prevent or mitigate some of the degenerative changes in mind and body so often blamed on aging. That includes the loss of the cells' electrical charges.

Since niacin is converted into niacinamide in the body, most vitamin B complex supplements, like enriched bread and flour, supply the vitamin in the form of niacinamide. There is another reason for choosing this form. If you were to ask a vitamin manufacturer what dictated the use of niacinamide rather than niacin, he would tell you that niacin causes flushing and a sensation of heat, which the public would not appreciate. Perhaps the public would, if they knew what you are about to learn: that the flush is the external token of an action of niacin, not yielded by niacinamide, which may help in avoiding heart and circulatory disorders.

Paradoxically, though the flush is listed as an action of niacin, it really isn't, at least not directly. If it were, you would have the experience every time you took the vitamin, which isn't always so. The increase in circulation comes indirectly, from the effect of niacin on "mast cells." These manufacture both histamine and a blood-thinner called heparin. The histamine causes the flush, and when repeated stimulation of its release from the mast cells has depleted the supply, the flush at least temporarily doesn't follow a niacin dose. The production of heparin is silent, yielding no perceptible symptoms, but in its own way it is even more potent a force in the body. The flushing from histamine is more than a nuisance, for its stimulation of circulation is used to help disorders in which circulation is compromised, like Raynaud's disease. But the production of heparin is another matter, for though it produces no flush or other overt reactions, it tends to lower blood fats, notably cholesterol and triglycerides, while helping circulation by easing the passage of red blood cells through the small blood vessels. Thus niacin, stimulating the release of heparin, duplicates some of the beneficial effects of the marine oils, discussed in Chapter 3.

Medicine has long known this action of niacin, for Dr. Edwin Boyle at the Miami Heart Institute long ago reported that there were 25 percent fewer nonfatal heart attacks in men treated with this form of the viatmin. The use of niacin was largely dropped, though, on the grounds that such massive doses were required that prohibitive side effects resulted. This, of course, is the logical outcome in a system of medicine oriented toward treatment rather than prevention. It overlooked, therefore, the possibility to which I direct your attention: the use of small amounts of niacin *before* circulation is compromised. It is very late to start when symptoms begin, for we have a 70 percent surplus of circulation, which means that matters are quite serious by the time we are down to the critical 30 percent, and suffering symptoms. With proper diet, always a prerequisite to the effective use of vitamins, minerals, and other supplements, niacin can be a friend to those who would conserve youth and well-being.

Remembering that successful therapy with nutrition is usually a monument to a lost opportunity for prevention, it is instructive to study what happens to middle-aged and elderly people, some of them senile, who are given niacin. In a long-ago book by one of my good friends, Dr. Abram Hoffer, a pioneer in orthomolecular psychiatry, he describes the responses of fifteen patients. Ten of these were senile, and of these, five recovered, two had marked improvement, and three did not respond. The action of niacin was not confined to the senile. The others slept better, had less fatigue, suffered fewer headaches, or commented on feeling more cheerful, happier, and more optimistic. It would be facile to credit these mood changes to a placebo effect, if it were not for an observation made by Dr. Tom Spies, who said he distinguished between thiamine (vitamin B_1) deficiency and niacin deficiency by telling the patient a funny story. If the patient laughed, the diagnosis of thiamine deficiency was confirmed, for lack of niacin extinguishes the sense of humor.

Other actions of the heparin response to niacin stimulation of the mast cells are all beneficial. Heparin tends to normalize blood cholesterol and triglycerides, lending support to the similar effects of the marine oils and of lecithin. A discussion of lecithin is found in Chapter 5.

After a lifetime of administering niacinamide to arthritics, one of my medical friends, Dr. William Kaufman, said this: "With this approach, we should have a new era of gerontology. It is even likely that certain aspects of what are today considered unavoidable consequences of the 'normal' aging process will disappear with the discovery and application of optimal nutrition in the management of an aging population. This is the hope for the future." The future has long been delayed, and I am about to take you into it, as we discuss what Dr. Kaufman accomplished with niacinamide in arthritis of the type usually blamed on aging, and, even more important, what he learned about preventing the joint disorders we blame on time.

In 1941, the physician began the use of niacinamide in his practice, beginning with certain types of neuropsychiatric and digestive disorders, which, he found, were corrected "rather promptly." He was fascinated when, in addition to other benefits, his patients reported decreased stiffness of joints. This directed the physician's attention to the possibility that old-age arthritis might be not only treated successfully with niacinamide, but prevented.

His results in treating osteoarthritis, which is the type linked medically with "wear and tear" and thereby with aging, were spectacular. As an example, he treated an aged woman with arthritis so severe that she was unable to leave her bed, brush her teeth, or comb her hair. Her joint mobility improved with niacinamide therapy to the point where she appeared in his office, neatly dressed, on her way to a church social, kissed him, and said: "You freed me from the prison of my arthritis." Other patients—not all, of course—reported increased alertness and decreased fatigability and irritability. The sense of well-being was heightened, and the appetite improved, as did muscle strength. Joint mobility improved, and, occasionally, joint deformities lessened. Not all patients were equally benefited by niacinamide treatment, and some experienced no subjective dividends such as increased well-being.

Dr. Kaufman identified certain organs and tissues as having a high requirement for niacinamide. These included muscles, movable joints, the membrane of the tongue, and that part of the spinal cord important to the function of the sense of balance. For those over fifty-five, he also listed certain parts of the brain. The reference to the sense of balance brings up the subject of an interesting test for niacinamide deficiency in the stages where it produces none of the symptoms classically attributed to it. With the eyes closed, the patient—always in the presence of an attendant, to avoid disastrous falling—is asked to raise his knee, clasping it so that the thigh is parallel with the floor. When this is done with the eyes closed, many patients with arthritis will tend to fall. Though niacinamide improves their sense of balance, that is not the point of this recital. In normal individuals, free of arthritis, the test may show impairment of the sense of balance, which means that the process which one day may result in osteoarthritis may be on its way. Restoration of that sense with sufficient dosage of niacinamide will eventuate in three months of treatment, if it is to occur. There is certainly an explicit lesson in this for those who seek old age with health unimpaired.

The lesson becomes more explicit, thanks to Dr. Kaufman's opportunity to apply niacinamide (and other B vitamins) preventively. He found that healthy people responded by not developing the joint stiffness usually blamed on old age—which is, of course, the moral to what you have read.

In the therapy for arthritis, this physician remarks, doses of niacinamide fifty to two hundred times the recommended dietary allowance can safely be prescribed for selected patients by supervising physicians. He warns that the mobility of the joints is affected *long* before the obvious evidence of arthritis appears. He stresses that the vitamin therapy will be effective only if the diet is adequate in protein and in calories. (The reason for the warning on calories is the tendency of the body to use protein needed for other purposes, as a source of calories when the diet doesn't supply enough.)

One patient's history beautifully illustrates what niacinamide may do in retarding degeneration usually attributed to growing old. A woman, fifty-two years of age, was treated for moderate joint dysfunction. In the third year of therapy, her moderate arthritis had literally disappeared, but she continued to take niacinamide for the next seventeen years, and the flexibility of her joints was that of "a healthy fifteen-year-old girl," and stayed at that level beyond her seventy-second year. She was taking 1,500 to 2,000 mg. of niacinamide daily.

If you're in your thirties or forties and free of impaired joint mobility and sense of balance, no such doses, which would call for medical supervision, would be needed. It is obvious, though, that 200 mg. daily would be a good investment: 100 mg. in the form of niacinamide, another 100 mg. in the form of niacin. The figure for niacin is tentative, for there are people, redheads particularly, who flush excessively and find the use of niacin intolerable. Others may find 100 mg. too high an intake. It is obvious that the vitamin investment, in both forms of niacin, is worthwhile for those who wish to keep joints and arteries young.

Based not only on Dr. Kaufman's findings—which I implicitly trust because he is both a physician and a Ph.D. in physiology—but also on my own long experience in the field of nutrition, let me note that the B vitamins are called a "complex" because they appear together in foods. This means that deficiency in only one of the B vitamins is unlikely. Not only are such deficiencies multiple, but these vitamins interlock in their physiological effects; hence taking them together makes sense. Your supplement of niacin and niacinamide, then, would be accompanied by a good vitamin B complex concentrate, a typical formula for which is described in Chapter 14.

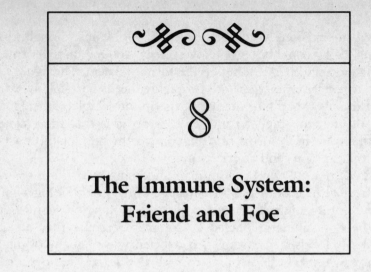

8

The Immune System:
Friend and Foe

Within us there is a complex and little-understood system of defense against bacteria, viruses, and cancer, called the immune system. Weakening of these defenses opens the door for degenerative disease and infections, serious enough in themselves, but also productive of changes in the body that we ordinarily blame on aging.

The immune system has been not only cavalierly neglected but actually abused in the practice of medicine, and the public has therefore been largely ignorant of its importance, except, perhaps, when publicity is given to children born with a genetic defect in the immune system, compelling them to live in plastic cocoons to avoid infections, which for them would be lethal, though for us merely inconveniences.

The immune system can be weakened by nutritional deficiencies, by drugs, by overdoses of nutrients, and by intense emotional disturbances. That explains the following discussion of pioneering research in immune-augmentation therapy for cancer, from which we can draw some conclusions about prevention. It also explains my recommendation of psychological counseling when you are faced with emotional crises beyond your capacity to bear. I mention this because those familiar with my dim view of psychiatry and psychoanalysis will otherwise think that I have ceased to endorse the philosophy of the Nobelist who stated that psychoanalysis will, like the auk, dodo, and dinosaur, leave no progeny. You have already read my criticism of psychiatric therapies when used on patients whose actual illness is physical rather than emotional or mental. Nonetheless, the psychiatrist can render yeoman service when we are helpless in the face of a catastrophic emotional storm.

Some twenty years ago, a researcher was seeking a natural substance in mouse blood that might stimulate the growth of cancer. That sounds paradoxical, but you can save time and money if your test animals don't take too long in developing the disease.

Dr. Lawrence Burton, a zoologist, found the factor he was seeking, but with it came something unexpected: an opposing substance in the blood that *retarded* the growth of animal cancer. This spurred him into decades of research in which he went ultimately from mouse to man, and arrived at a cancer treatment, often successful, using factors normal to human blood.

This scientist's work taught us a great deal about the immune system. Not only had he identified previous unknown immune factors that, perhaps every day, stamp out cancer in the healthy, but he gave us a view, for the first time, of the influence of the emotions on the immune system.

Dr. Burton found but four immune factors, of the possible hundreds, the ratios among which determine whether cancer gains headway or is extirpated. Briefly, these consist of tumor complement, tumor antibody, blocking protein (which defends the cancer and is also produced by it), and deblocking protein, which cancels some of the effects of the blocker. When cancer is present, these factors are usually imbalanced, and by adjusting the ratios, each to each, striking control of cancer, even in terminal patients, has been attained. So much for the theory of the treatment. Functioning in healthy people, one would expect to find normal ratios of these chemicals of immunity. Not so: Dr. Burton informed me that there are those yet in good health whose immune factors are nonetheless out of balance. These people he regards as on the way toward cancer, and good subjects for prevention.

I asked Dr. Burton about the condition of the immune systems of newly arrived cancer patients, expecting him to tell me that there were serious deficiencies of the factors of immunity. "Not so," he said. "When they first arrive, they are optimistic, for someone is going to do something to help them, and that emotion buoys the immune system. A few days later, when they realize that, yes, someone is helping, but they still have cancer and their lives are still threatened, the bottom falls out of the immune system." Expanding on the role of the emotions in immune functions, he added, "If the patient is hit by a virus during the treatment, we lose him. The immune system can't take care of two significant insults at once. And the insults don't have to be infections. They can be emotional. I nearly lost a woman," he reminisced, "who was responding beautifully to the therapy, when she received a letter from her husband, telling her that he was unable to bear the expense and the strain of her illness, and that he wanted a divorce. Her immune system dropped sharply, even though we increased the doses of the factors, and the cancer gained headway."

I thought of those remarks when I read a paper on an experiment in which physicians made prophecies for the survival time of terminal cancer patients. The oncologists did if after careful examination. Psychiatrists did it without seeing the patients, basing their predictions on psychological descriptions of the sufferers. Yet the psychiatrists were as accurate as the cancer specialists in estimating remaining length of life. This confirms an ancient observation which credits optimistic cancer sufferers with longer survival than the despondent who passively surrender to the disease.

The role of the emotions in supporting or depressing the immune system was explored in a study at New York's Mount Sinai Hospital, which revealed a threatening collapse of the immune system in men who had lost their wives to breast cancer. This explained the startlingly high mortality and morbidity rates in widowers, many of whom suffer cancer, a devastating heart attack, or other life-threatening disease within two years after bereavement. If you wonder why I specify men, it's because women are blessed genetically with a more vigorous immune system that more effectively protects widows.

As one of the authorities on stress, Dr. Paul Rosch, has said, it is evident that the brain has conversations with the immune system, and we may hope that one day we'll learn how to eavesdrop on those exchanges, and modify their effects when necessary for our benefit. From research reported at the American Institute of Stress, we can already demonstrate in animals that the immune system and the brain are linked, even at the level of a simple conditioned reflex. A striking experiment showed that rats given an indigestion-producing drug, and simultaneously given sweetened water, ultimately conditioned the stimulus, so that gastric cramps were produced by the sweetened water alone, without the drug. By chance, the medication used to produce intestinal symptoms also depressed the immune system. When the response was conditioned, so that the sweetened water alone produced cramps, it also lowered the activity of the immune system. Here was a clear-cut demonstration of interaction between brain and nervous systems, and the body's arsenal of defense.

You may not have thought so as I have guided you through this maze, but surely you now realize that bottling the impact of overwhelming stress is a direct attack on the body's system of defenses, vital both to health and normal aging. When the stress is intolerable, you need catharsis. The listening ear is critical, and some experience in counseling obviously necessary, but your outlet need not be a psychiatrist or psychologist. It can be a minister, priest, rabbi, or social worker, anyone with experience who will listen and not sit in judgment.

Medicine's view of the immune system has been myopic. I'm not complaining about the failure to appreciate the importance of factors of immunity, nor about the prescription of drugs that depress the system, healing one illness but inviting another. I am not faulting physicians for what they didn't know, for hindsight is usually 20/20. But when you understand the immune system, even to the limited extent that we do, and look back at medical practices in the past fifty years, it appears as if the profession had an animosity against the factors that protect us against invaders.

For example, the thymus gland, which is a mainspring of our immunities, was deliberately shrunk with irradiation years ago. They had compared the thymus glands of infants with those of adults, and found the babies' glands to be so much larger that they considered them hypertrophied (overgrown), and therefore used irradiation to shrink them. However, the "normal" adult thymus, used as a model, was usually taken from the corpse of a patient who had died with a wasting disease, and in such illnesses, the thymus shrinks dramatically. Thereby, this, the gland central to a baby's resistance to invaders, was ignorantly attacked. It should be noted that even in healthy adults, the thymus gland shrinks as age accumulates. This may explain the lowered resistance of the elderly to some infections, which for them (and not for younger people) may be life threatening. This should call to mind the warnings by health departments, in epidemics of influenza, that the elderly especially need immunizing injections.

Removal of the appendix is perhaps the most common surgical maneuver in this country, and only recently was it realized that this "atavistic" organ with no apparent function except to enrich surgeons actually plays a part in the immune system. This might explain some of the allergic reactions patients experience after appendectomies, sometimes for the first time in their lives.

Still another insult was another common type of surgery, the tonsillectomy. This operation was considered so minor that it actually was performed in physicians' offices, sometimes on the slender justification of repeated "sore throats." Experience showed that the operation reduced the frequency and severity of attacks of tonsillitis, but increased the incidence of more serious respiratory infections. This was interpreted as meaning that the tonsils constitute a barrier that is *supposed* to become infected, thereby intercepting the bacteria that otherwise would invade the lungs or cause bronchitis. Actually, the significance was greater than that, for it was learned, once again, that the tonsils are part of the complex immune system. Indeed, the medical journals were filled with reports that those whose tonsils had been removed were more prone to polio, of the severest type, and to a type of cancer.

While the immune system was being physically debilitated, it was (and is) being weakened by dietary deficiencies, many of them the result of food processing as well as the consumer's ignorance of the criteria of good nutrition. The removal of zinc, manganese, and selenium from foods was excused when these nutrients were not recognized as essential to human beings. However, recognition didn't stop the mills from grinding, because the industry promptly took refuge in the doctrine that we don't live by bread, rice, or corn alone, and their deficits could be offset by nutrient contributions from other foods. The problem was that the processors of the other foods used the same excuse. One is reminded of independent contractors, each building a separate piling to support a bridge, and each excusing his use of inferior concrete on the grounds that the bridge doesn't depend on *his* piling alone.

A lifetime of diet low in the factors needed for immunity is serious enough, but it acts as an added insult, for the immune system loses efficiency as the years accrue. Good nutrition may not cancel but certainly would slow the time-associated drop in immune functions. Recognition of that interrelationship is now finding its way into the publications of orthodox institutions, which a few years ago would have summarily rejected the thesis. So we find Sloan Kettering publishing a paper, for example, on failure of the immune system when zinc intake is inadequate, as it is for many Americans. (On the other hand, consider the implications of the controversy between Dr. Linus Pauling and the cancer researchers of the Mayo Clinic, which I discussed on page 71.)

There are companies that sell desiccated thymus tissue, while avoiding claims for its stimulating effect on the immune system. I have reservations about the usefulness of such supplements, for the same reason that makes eating sweetbreads (actually, thymus glands) a futile effort to influence the immune system. The process of digestion of protein will almost certainly break down the intricate linkages of amino acids comprising the thymus hormones. I am a little ambivalent, though, for the orthodoxy says the same thing about pancreatic enzymes, which are also protein and also theoretically broken down in the digestive processes; and yet I have seen therapeutic responses to treatment with pancreatin, though it had to be given in tremendous doses.

However, there is a mineral nutrient that has a potent stimulating effect on the thymus gland. Oddly enough, I do not find manganese listed among such nutrients in popular books, however erudite, on nutrition. Yet years ago, a specialist in myasthenia gravis (grave weakening of the muscles) found thymus atrophy to be linked with the disease, and reported that manganese treatment had actually reversed the shrinkage, restoring the gland almost to normal size. This action of the nutrient has apparently been forgotten, but with involution of the thymus as we age, lowering our resistance to aging itself and the disorders concomitant with it, we should have a keen interest in maintaining manganese intake. The germ or bran of the grain tends to concentrate manganese, but processing depletes those values, and so does the common method of fertilization, for liming of the soil increases foliage but decreases the manganese level of the vegetable crop. The organ meats, like liver, are a good source, but protein foods otherwise are not.

Emphasis has been placed on the stabilizing effect of manganese on cell membranes, critically important to some epileptics, but also to the rest of us, for this action makes manganese important to avoid excessive nerve irritability. Manganese is also a stimulant to the pituitary gland, as is PABA. Animals deprived of the mineral have no maternal instinct, refuse to nurse their young, and allow them to die. Since we have a vested interest in maintaining pituitary function, we have another reason to guard our manganese intake, which should be in the neighborhood of 4 mg. daily, assuming adequate reserves, which would mean a long history of eating whole grains in preference to milled carbohydrates. If the dietary history isn't virtuous, we may bring up the reserves by supplementing the diet with 25 mg. daily. Those with high blood pressure who take more than 4 or 5 mg. daily should do so under medical direction, for idiosyncrasy of reaction may elevate the pressure more.

For some women, manganese shares with zinc an action that reduces the tendency to depression in the premenstrual week. In some instances, there is an elevation of blood copper levels at that time. Both manganese and zinc have an anticopper effect, which then becomes useful.

I have mentioned that American zinc reserves are so low that a single day of fasting may be memorialized later by the appearance of white spots on the nails as they grow. The metal is vital to the prostate gland, which, desiccated, actually contains 50 percent zinc. This concentration explains the use of zinc and vitamin B_6, which aids in its absorption, in the treatment of the benign enlarged prostate, a condition common in older men, and considerably uncomfortable. This therapeutic application certainly suggests that this common male disorder may be mitigated, if not prevented, by adequate intake of zinc, which many of us don't achieve, and of vitamin B_6, which, you have learned, we similarly neglect. Meanwhile, the vitamin may be helping you to avoid atherosclerosis, and the zinc will be supporting your immune system, which it markedly stimulates, as well as lending help in avoiding atherosclerosis.

Though physicians in therapeutic indications may use much more, 15 mg. of zinc is probably the most popular supplementary dose. Be careful to read the label, if you buy the supplement, for the total weight of the zinc compound is greater than the amount of elemental zinc it supplies.

The foods rich in zinc are whole barley, beef, beets, carrots, whole corn, egg yolk, liver, oatmeal, peas, brown rice, whole wheat, and wheat bran. Oysters are a rich source, but may present a risk of excessive amounts of cadmium. This good food is also sometimes contaminated with the hepatitis virus.

Vitamin C is intimately involved in the function of the immune system. It concentrates in the outer area of white blood cells, which are part of our security force against invasion by bacteria, viruses, and cancer. Interferon, hailed as but certainly *not* the significant cancer preventive or treatment among the discoveries of this century, is but one of our factors of immunity against such invaders, and the production of interferon is increased by vitamin C. The vitamin is intimately involved in the processes by which the body gets rid of excess cholesterol, a finding demonstrated in rabbits as well as human beings. It is interesting that the animals manufacture their vitamin C, and yet profit by high-potency supplements, equivalent in terms of human body weight to something like 7,500 mg. (7.5 grams) of the vitamin daily. The ideal amount of the vitamin differs from person to person, the range of requirement being between 250 mg. and 2,500 mg. daily. One criterion of excessive intake, in terms of individual requirement, is excessive laxative effect. While I am not impressed with the claims made for time-release supplements, because the technique too often doesn't work, I have found time-release vitamin C useful. This allows lower dosage, while maintaining blood levels better than intermittent intake of the vitamin in its usual form. Queried about vitamin C requirements, and not speaking in terms of the huge doses used in the treatment of hepatitis and other serious disease, Dr. Linus Pauling responded interestingly, saying that man, if he could synthesize the vitamin like most other animals, would be manufacturing about 2,500 mg. daily. In the face of potent stress, again assuming man's ability to synthesize at the rate of lower animals, man might manufacture 10,000 mg. daily.

Most of us know that the citrus fruits are rich sources of

vitamin C. Few realize that there is an accompanying nutrient in these and other vitamin C sources. These are the bioflavonoids, important to our blood vessels and protectors of vitamin C against the degrading effects of oxygen in the body. The bioflavonoids are largely removed when orange juice is strained, and brands which contain pulp are recommended. Orange juice in paper cartons loses vitamin C very rapidly, making glass-packed juice a better choice. Despite the emphasis on citrus fruits, there are numerous other foods that fortify our vitamin C intake, including broccoli, cauliflower, collards, kale, mustard greens, green peppers, strawberries, and turnip greens. If you don't want to revive the old phrase "throwing the baby out with the bathwater," it is imperative to minimize cooking water and to save and use it for soups, gravies, and sauces, for it is often astonishingly high in vitamin C value.

In the discussion of antioxidants (Chapter 5) it became obvious that some of the effects we attribute to vitamin E deficiency actually result from the toxic action of oxygen on unsaturated (vegetable) fats in the body. However, an unappreciated dividend from adequate vitamin E intake is stimulation of the immune system, which is dramatic only when dosage is high, so high that the effect appears more pharmacological (druglike) than nutritional. The effective doses for the animals should not, without testing in human beings, be transferred to man. However, it certainly makes sense for the average American to use supplements of the vitamin in the amounts described (see page 56) and to increase the intake of foods with generous values in the vitamin. Despite assurances that we Americans need have no concern about vitamin E intake, an examination at Tulane Medical School of a random sample of American adults showed a large majority with the biochemical stigmata of vitamin E deficiency. From what you have already read, this dietary error promotes rapid aging and is a threat to arteries, heart, and the immune mechanism. Many nutritionists, including me, regard the standard for dietary intake of vitamin E to be entirely too low. This level certainly didn't take into consideration the latter-day fad for increased consumption of polyunsaturated fats, which raises vitamin E requirement by an order of magnitude. Indeed, the standard of intake for many animals, ranging from chickens to rats, is about five times that for human beings.

The standard textbooks claim a comfortable content of vitamin E in vegetable oils. This should not be taken at face value, for I know of at least one major producer who removes the vitamin from the oil, sells it to the vitamin industry, who sell it back to the consumers who buy the oil. Ironically, we need six-tenths of a milligram of vitamin E to protect a gram of vegetable fat from oxidation in the body, a protective effect critical to slowing down aging. In the charts, margarine is listed as a rich source, but you will later learn that an abnormal type of fat created in the partial hydrogenation of the fat in margarine is toxic, and conducive to some of the ills we blame on aging. Other than the purported vitamin E value of the vegetable oils, useful amounts of vitamin E are yielded by whole grains, wheat germ, and wheat germ oil. (Note that peanut oil, which has undesirable characteristics, is also a very poor source of vitamin E.) Wheat germ oil has a strong flavor, so it is best used by combining it with your preferred salad oils. When you buy such oils, be sure that they do not contain butyl hydroxytoluene (BHT) or butyl hydroxyanisole (BHA). These are antioxidants, preservatives, originally formulated to protect the colors in motion picture film from fading. Though used in a thousand foods in this country, their use—particularly BHT—has been banned outright or the quantities severely limited or the use restricted to a few foods in several countries; and the World Health Organization pronounced BHT to be so dangerous that its use in baby foods was disapproved. When you read eulogies of these synthetic antioxidants, or recommendation of their ingestion by human beings, it may be rewarding to check the associations of the nutritionist with the chemical industry.

Selenium, which has a biochemical partnership with vitamin E, is another nutrient specifically important to the immune system. It is also an antioxidant. It has both an anticarcinogenic effect and an anti-aging action. Unknown to the public and, largely, to the medical profession, is research at a veterans' hospital in which chemotherapy, usually unsuccessful in lung cancer, was fortified with large doses of selenium, the combined treatment proving to be remarkably more effective than the drug therapy alone. Significant is the amount of selenium in human milk, about six times as much as in cow's milk. (The vitamin E value is twice as high.)

Good food sources of selenium are eggs (because the chickens receive supplements to keep them healthy), brewer's yeast, liver, and most foods of animal origin. The comparatively low values of vegetable foods indicate that vegetarians should be using yeast supplements. Grain products lose varying amounts of selenium in processing. White bread has lost 50 percent. White rice has one-fifteenth the quantity of selenium in brown rice. With its importance to the protection of the immune system, deriving from its antioxidant effects, and the protection it offers for the genetic messages in our cells, selenium is a long-neglected, much-maligned nutrient that deserves your attention.

The thymus gland has another nutritional protector: vitamin A, which also stimulates the immune system and protects us against some of the cancer-causing agents in our environment. While the arena of nutrition has been discordant with cries of toxicity of this vitamin, surveys over and over again show that millions of Americans don't consume the modest requirement of the vitamin set by the recommended dietary allowances. Oddly, vitamin A and its precursor in foods, beta carotene, seem to act individually as anticarcinogens. This makes intake of leafy vegetables, and carrots, for carotene, as important as consumption of sources of preformed vitamin A, such as liver, whole milk, and butter. From what you have learned about the value of the marine oils in protecting our arteries, it should be obvious that old-fashioned cod liver oil, supplying EPA and DHA as well as vitamins A and D, has virtues not provided by the vitamin A and D concentrates used in modern vitamin supplements.

Vitamin A should not be described as toxic. Toxicity is a property of dose, and overdosage of anything, including water, is toxic. Adequately provided by the diet or supplements, the vitamin increases longevity, delays senility, and at the same time helps the immune system. Good food sources of carotene include apricots, beet greens, broccoli, cantaloupe, chard, kale, spinach, sweet potatoes, and turnip greens. Liver is a superb source of preformed vitamin A. In fact, even a serving of liver once a week serves as a vitamin A insurance policy. The form of liver the public prefers is, as usual, the least valuable: calf's liver. The mature animal has had more time to build up vitamin A stores. Pork, lamb, and beef liver are therefore more valuable. I might note that there is what amounts to a superstition that liver is a concentrated source of the pesticides and insecticides that contaminate our environment. Assays I have examined do not confirm that.

There are amino acids that increase thymus weight and stimulate the immune system. I am wary of the use of individual amino acids without expert medical supervision. I am aware that arginine, recommended by some authors in my field, blocks the formation of some tumors, but I'm also aware that higher arginine intake may be an invitation to a herpes infection. At the moment, at least, I prefer the safety of the amino acids supply as it comes to us in such efficient protein sources as eggs, meat, fish, fowl, and most of the dairy products.

Animal research suggests that protein-digesting enzymes also stimulate segments of the immune system. These include trypsin, bromelain (from uncooked pineapple), and papain (from the papaya fruit and seeds). There is another rationale for using these enzyme preparations, which are available in health food stores, with the exception of trypsin. My experience with the elderly has convinced me that both hydrochloric acid production and the digestive enzyme supply are progressively less adequate in the aging. The health food stores sell betaine hydrochloride as a precursor of the stomach's manufacture of hydrochloric acid. From the physician's point of view, the results are less than satisfactory, but the use of bromelain and papain has been helpful to digestion in many of the aging. In addition to the digestive effect of bromelain, it also stimulates the production of a hormone, prostaglandin E_1, a short supply of which can contribute to a host of disorders, ranging from atopic eczema to premenstrual tension. The use of moderate amounts of these enzymes for their beneficial effect on the immune system makes sense. Their use for their effect on efficiency of digestion, though, is rational only when one's utilization of protein foods is inefficient. Not incidentally, I should remind you that utilization of protein tends to diminish as the years accrue, and vitamin B_6 (pyridoxine) helps to offset that effect.

There are sulfur compounds that markedly stimulate the immune system, one of them, ironically, provided most richly by the eggs they tell us not to eat. Garlic supplies a useful form of sulfur, which may be responsible for its beneficial effect on hypertension. Cysteine, which is an amino acid containing sulfur, also stimulates the immune system. It is a sulfur source in eggs, and I prefer to use it that way because of my reservations on unsupervised self-dosage with individual amino acids. As an example of my reservations, consider that methionine, another amino acid, is a good source of sulfur, but if taken without vitamin B_6, you have learned, it may contribute to atherosclerosis. In susceptible individuals, methionine produces a feeling of depersonalization or detachment from reality. All told, your amino acids are more acceptable (and certainly taste better) when procured from steak, eggs, liver, and other good animal protein foods. I emphasize animal protein as a source of sulfur as I do animal foods as sources of selenium, and the same warning emerges for vegetarians: if you don't at least eat eggs, you may be sulfur-deficient. And if the cholesterol phobia is still with you, even after reading this book, consider that two eggs daily raise blood cholesterol by only *2 percent,* certainly not enough to threaten your arteries. Once again, I have a subterranean thought overriding what I have written. Nobody seems to know that the American Cancer Society studied the effect of eating (or not eating) eggs on the life span. Some 200,000 subjects were in each group. The egg-eaters outlived the egg-avoiders by a significant margin. Perhaps more efficient immune systems made for the difference.

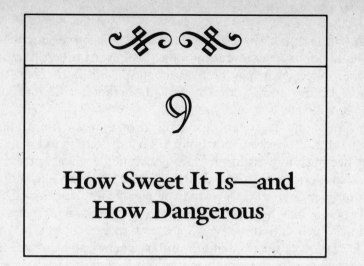

9

How Sweet It Is—and How Dangerous

Browsing through a medical journal rather than the outdated magazines in your physician's waiting room, the odds are that you'd pass by an advertisement of a self-test for blood sugar levels in diabetics. Yet that advertisement makes statements of great importance to you. One of those is: "An improved quality of life and improved psychological well-being are dividends from monitoring of blood sugar." Without self-monitoring, and, I hope, without diabetes, that statement is of vital importance to you, because disturbances of the body's management of sugar (and starch) are pathways to serious troubles, and, indeed, may be symptomatic of underlying and threatening major disorders.

Reflect on the fact that when diabetics are examined carefully, heart disease and atherosclerosis are frequently found. Conversely, when patients with heart disease and hardening of the arteries are carefully examined, diabetes, full-fledged or incipient, is frequently found. One doesn't have to be a medical genius to decide that this evidence points to a cause common to all these disorders. It may not be the only one; it may be but a predisposing factor, but disturbances of the body's control of carbohydrates are warnings to change your life-style and your diet.

Examining the sugar content of a drop of blood is not a test for disturbed carbohydrate metabolism. That drop of blood is a mirror of a fleeting moment in physiological time; as such, it may show elevated blood sugar (or a deficiency in it) but nothing more. At that moment, the sugar level may be normal in that drop of blood, and yet you may be a victim of deranged carbohydrate metabolism and, as such, faced with a very real threat to health, to the prolongation of the time of life, and to an enjoyable old age.

The body, with its built-in wisdom (homeostasis), manages to keep itself on an even keel in the midst of forces of anarchy. It releases stored sugar when an emergency makes physical demands upon its energy reserves. Lacking enough carbohydrate (starch and sugar) to meet its requirements, it will change fuels, and burn fat for energy. With insufficient protein in the diet, it will, if compelled, tear down its own protein structures, to distribute the supply more equitably. But there are insults where the wisdom of the body must fail. Among these are excess intake of certain types of food that nature never made available, and inadequacies in the supplies of external factors the body needs to metabolize foods. These problems, common in civilization, are intensified as the organism ages, its wisdom dilutes, and it loses some of its ability to create enzymes and other factors vital to its chemistries. These are, of course, problems at any age level, but increasingly frequent as we age. Since, in essence, they create malnutrition, sometimes in the midst of plenty, they are also conducive to premature aging, for the symptoms of long-term malnourishment match (and intensify) those we blame on aging.

The physician is understandably reluctant to order the test needed to evaluate glucose tolerance, because it takes six hours (sometimes eight hours) and is both inconvenient and expensive. No one enjoys six or more withdrawals of blood, and many hours in the testing laboratory. Yet this is indispensable in appraising carbohydrate metabolism, for in the test, the body is challenged with what the professional considers a large dose of glucose (sugar). The irony of it is apparent when I tell you that many Americans take that much sugar in foods and beverages, sometimes in the morning hours alone, thereby giving themselves a "sugar challenge." After determining the fasting blood sugar level and giving the challenge dose, the physician will then sample blood sugar levels at intervals for the duration of the test. Frequently, the level is normal at one blood withdrawal and totally abnormal in another, which explains why the one-drop-of-blood technique can give a false assurance of all being well.

In some people, about 5 percent of the population, the body reacts to the challenge with grossly elevated blood sugar. In others, perhaps 10 to 20 percent of the population, the sugar challenge elevates the blood sugar, but not high enough, or causes the level to drop (reactive hypoglycemia); in still others, there is a normal rise, but it not only isn't normally sustained, but is followed by a drop below the level needed to maintain mental and physical functions. This is low blood sugar.

While in this discussion we are concerned with avoiding the dietary mistakes and the life-style that disturb carbohydrate metabolism, I have discussed this test because I think it important that it be included in your medical checkups, and the reasons for that are obvious.

I have referred repeatedly to the mischief created by excessive intake of sugar, indicting it for excessive stimulation of stomach acid activity, increase in platelet adhesiveness, boosting blood cholesterol and triglyceride levels, and, something I didn't mention before, stimulating the undesirable release of free fatty acids at the aorta. Human beings being human, you exonerated yourself from the sin of eating too much sugar and mentally promised to tell George or Kathy about its dangers. But the average consumption of sugar is 120 pounds a year, the figure from which I derive my statement that you, as an average American, manage to swallow a teaspoonful of the stuff every thirty-five minutes, twenty-four hours a day. When you deny that because you don't eat candy, you fall into the trap of hidden sugar, which is in the form in which the bulk of the intake enters the diet. Ketchup is one-fifth sugar, and it's your fault, because the manufacturers, who used to make the product less sweet, found it sold better with more sugar. A doughnut is five teaspoonfuls. So is a small bottle of soda pop. Salad dressing contains sugar; even salt sometimes does, for dextrose, which is sugar, is used as an anticaking agent. Ice cream is 16 percent sugar.

There is sweetening in your cough medicine and in the antacid tablets you use (for the indigestion caused by too much sugar). Shake 'n Bake is 50 percent sugar. Breakfast cereals contain large amounts. Apple pie supplies twelve teaspoonfuls of sugar per slice; cherry pie, fourteen. Embellish that with ice cream, as many people who like pie à la mode do, and you have eighteen or more teaspoonfuls of sugar per portion. Every sugar crystal requires thiamine (B_1), niacinamide, and chromium to metabolize it, and sugar supplies none of these factors. That means that your sweet tooth deprives you of critically important factors in retarding aging, increasing the need while decreasing the supply.

All this leads inevitably to a simple conclusion, which I'm going to capitalize:

SHARPLY REDUCING YOUR SUGAR INTAKE IS URGENT.

From what you've read, avoiding the sugar bowl isn't enough. The ubiquitous use of sugar in the manufacture of processed foods, condiments, beverages, and desserts makes it important to read the ingredient list on food labels. Even then, you can be deceived if you are not familiar with the devices that manufacturers, well aware of rising public antipathy to high-sugar foods, use to lull you into obliviousness. Ordinarily, the ingredients are listed in the percentage order of their presence, so that sugar, if the main ingredient, would appear first on the list. You find it's fourth, let's say, but don't stop there. Two lines below is listed dextrose or glucose, and a line below that, corn syrup solids. Those are all sugar, and in large quantities they are undesirable. If they were lumped together, sugar might indeed be the major ingredient. Read labels carefully. If you don't, just as an example, you can bring home yogurt that has more calories from sugar than it does from the life-supporting nutrients you are entitled to expect from a dairy product.

I have already told you that sugar increases the need for the vitamin B complex while not supplying these vitamins. Remember that deficiency in these factors, particularly when it is mild and chronic, causes changes in the body, the skin, and the mind which are often indistinguishable from those we have attributed to aging. Even as I wrote that sentence, I was thinking of an elderly woman who had complained to her doctor that she always felt "swimmy-headed." He happened to remember that Dr. Tom Spies had described that feeling as characteristic of patients with early symptoms of pellagra, and gave the patient doses of niacinamide. She returned with the physical benefits later reported by Dr. William Kaufman, but she also said that for the first time in many years she was able to think clearly. I could multiply by a thousand stories and case histories parallel with that, and the result would be a fragment of the experiences that emphasize the importance of a diet low in sugar, high in vitamin B complex, and supplemented with a concentrate of the B vitamins as dietary insurance. Later in this chapter, you will find a list of foods rich in these vitamins.

Even textbooks currently in use in university nutrition courses have little to say about deficiency in chromium, for the research is too recent to be acceptable. Yet that research clearly indicates that chromium is essential to carbohydrate metabolism, and that the body steadily loses the ability to convert the metal into the complex form in which it is utilized. Added to that, not only has sugar parted with its chromium in the processing, but it increases the excretion of the nutrient. Still other research shows that a deficiency of the chromium glucose tolerance (CGT) factor can cause a mild type of diabetes, particularly in the aged. Other studies indicate that the CGT factor is beneficial to younger diabetics, reducing their need for insulin. The metal itself is used by the body only in the form of the glucose tolerance factor, in which it is a part of a complex molecule, which contains, among other entities, niacinamide. It is failure to form this compound, rather than deficiency in chromium, then, which is our concern. This makes use of the preformed factor, rather than metallic chromium, a sound nutritional practice. Yeast that has been concentrated for its content of the CGT factor is now available, a typical brand yielding 15 mcg. of organically bound chromium per tablet. The usual recommendation is 30 mcg. (two tablets) daily for those under forty years of age, and double that for those over forty.

Vitamin B complex supplements sometimes appear to have been formulated by a bookkeeper rather than a nutritionist, containing generous amounts of factors that are inexpensive and lip-service amounts of others. A typical example is a formula with a very long list of ingredients, containing only 2 mcg. of chromium as the CGT factor, large amounts of thiamine and other B vitamins, but only 5 mg. of PABA and 100 mg. of choline. The chromium,

PABA, and choline might just as well have been omitted, as the quantities are too small to supply any real dietary insurance. In Chapter 14, I outline the type of formula that makes more sense.

Meanwhile, it also makes sense to select foods that are good sources of the vitamin B complex. Though these vitamins tend to appear together, some foods are richer in a given factor than others, and diversification of your choices is intelligent. Generally speaking, organ meats such as liver, grains that are unprocessed, and brewer's yeast are good choices. Pork is an excellent source of thiamine, as are peas, pecans, soybeans, wheat germ, kidney and lima beans, and oatmeal—the last being probably the best choice in cooked cereals, all values considered.

Riboflavin, important to eyesight, skin, blood, and the nervous system, is richly provided by liver, milk, heart, Cheddar cheese, and almonds.

Niacin, properties of which you have encountered, is found in almonds, beef, fish, peanuts and peanut butter (richly), tuna, pork, whole grains, liver, and wheat germ. The diet deficient in this factor is often deficient in protein, for the protein (amino) acid tryptophane is used by the body as a precursor of synthesis of niacinamide.

Vitamin B_6 (pyridoxine), which I have described as a possible preventive of atherosclerosis, is possibly important to our skin and definitely vital to blood-forming tissues and to the brain and nervous system. In the elderly, it is helpful in the utilization of protein, sometimes offsetting the tendency of the aged to excrete more protein (nitrogen) than they are ingesting. Bananas are a rich source, and liver, once again; peas, halibut, lettuce, beef, peanuts, both Irish and sweet potatoes, pork, and wheat germ are good sources.

Inositol, deficiency of which encourages the nervous-system complications of diabetes, and which is involved in fat and cholesterol metabolism, is richly provided by beef brain, heart, and liver, and comes to you in cantaloupe, oranges, peanuts, raisins, Irish and sweet potatoes, strawberries, and whole grains, with wheat germ again a very good source.

Biotin, essential to our skin, heart, and energy metabolism, is synthesized in the body by intestinal bacteria, making deficiency improbable, though it occasionally is reported. The foods supplying it have already been listed as supplying other B vitamins.

Folic acid, requisite to blood formation and to the nervous system, is richly provided by liver, peanuts, whole wheat, wheat germ, many green, leafy vegetables, bananas, mushrooms, Irish potatoes, and salmon.

Choline, important to the liver, vital to the functioning of the brain and the muscles, kidneys, and eyes, is outstandingly provided by eggs (yolks), soybeans, corn and wheat germ, whole wheat, spinach, oats, peanuts and peanut butter, peas, and kidneys.

The vitamin B complex, comprising this entire group of vitamins, including a number of factors known to exist but not yet chemically identified, was best described by Dr. Tom Spies, the medical nutritionist whom I have quoted previously. He said: "Exclusive of ascorbic acid, it is a composite of all the water-soluble vitamins found in yeast and liver. Included among the vitamins is a heterogeneous conglomeration of compounds whose structures differ greatly, and whose functions, as far as known, differ even more. Their common features are that they are not built up by the body, at least in the amount needed, and that they carry on their several functions when present in small concentration or only in traces."

Perhaps what you have read lends credence to several facets of my nutritional philosophy. You can understand now why I take a dim view of diets, like the low-cholesterol, which forbid consumption of liver and tend to inhibit the use of milk and dairy products. You can also understand why we nutritionists place so much emphasis on protecting your intake of the vitamin B complex, and so invidiously criticize the food processors for removing this group of vitamins from your food. What you have read will emphasize the importance of using natural sources of vitamin B complex, both in the diet and in supplements, to provide protective amounts not only of the known B vitamins, but of the many factors as yet unidentified. No one knows the identity of the antifatigue factor in liver, but with fatigue the most common complaint brought to physicians, in the absence of disease, is not use of more liver in the diet, and desiccated liver as a supplement, rational?

With that next spoonful of sugar, that sugar-filled confection, that bottle of soda pop, will you reflect on what you are doing? You are increasing your need for the B vitamins while lowering the supply. It is a game that yields no prizes.

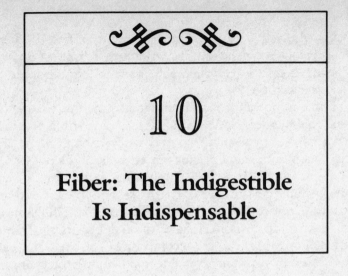

10

Fiber: The Indigestible Is Indispensable

It takes but a few hours of watching television to realize that constipation is the problem of millions of Americans, who yield to electronic persuasion by purchasing some 200 million dollars' worth of laxatives, lubricants, suppositories, and enema paraphernalia yearly. Both physicians and the public regarded the difficulty as just that, a small problem with a facile if temporary remedy. The complications of chronic constipation, including hemorrhoids and fistulas, were dealt with by surgery. Other complications were not recognized as such, including diverticulosis, diverticulitis, appendicitis, thrombosis of the deep veins, hiatus hernia, and bowel cancer.

The relationship between a low-fiber diet and these disorders was recognized, long after it should have been, because of the pioneering research of an English physician who was puzzled by the obvious immunity of Central Africans to these "complications of constipation" and to constipation itself. He found the answer in the fiber intake of these primitives, though the difference between theirs and ours is only a few grams daily. Those few grams, though, can be the difference between glowing health and a long list of dismal disorders. Very significant is the fact that the disorders I listed above are so rare in Central Africans that cases of them are regarded as medical curiosities, in sharp contrast to our vast population of sufferers. When an African does develop one of these disasters, the odds are great that he deserted his ancestral diet and was seduced by the convenience of Western foods.

Insufficient fiber intake is behind two disturbances of which we were not aware, or which we considered unimportant. One of these is slow stool transit time. The other is a concomitant bacterial attack on food residues that linger in the colon too long. Slow transit time for the residues of food is a concept that people tend to resist if they are not constipated. It has nothing to do with frequency of bowel movement. One may have an evacuation every day and still be a victim of slow stool transit time. Perhaps the easiest way to explain it is to say that the regular bowel movement that occurred on Sunday should have eventuated the day before, or even two days before. This delay allows the bacteria in the bowel a chance, at their leisure, to break down chemicals normal to the stool, converting them into carcinogens (cancer-causing agents) of great and deadly potency. The result of chronic slow transit time, then, is years of bathing the delicate tissues of the bowel in carcinogenic agents. This is held responsible for bowel cancer, high on the list of the deadly forms of the disease, and so common in the United States that there are "colostomy clubs" of survivors, united to help newcomers to adjust to the postsurgical trauma of the condition.

The bacteria that attack the food residues in the bowel are considered the "unfriendly" type, for obvious reasons. Therefore, increasing fiber intake to decrease stool transit time is not enough. An effort must be made to replace the hostile bacteria with beneficial types. Many individuals attempt to use yogurt for that purpose, although the amount needed for effectiveness would be prohibitive. It is more promising to fortify yogurt with lactobacillus bacteria, which are available freeze-dried, in capsules, whose contents can be mixed with yogurt. When you buy yogurt, I should add, avoid those with added sugar, jam, preserves, and additives. A fine yogurt will contain nothing but milk, low- or full-fat, and the bacterial culture. Commercial yogurt is equivalent to buying milk at five dollars per gallon or thereabouts, and it is sensible to make your own. A yogurt maker, which is simply a low-heat hot plate, is inexpensive, and adding the bacterial culture is simple. You inoculate the milk with a few teaspoonfuls of any good, plain yogurt. In adding the capsulated freeze-dried bacterial culture, use the amount (per cup of yogurt) specified on the label as a daily supplement.

The two most effective forms of fiber are bran and carrots, cooked or uncooked. Carrot fiber yields a stool of ice-cream consistency, eliminating the need for pressure in evacuation, and thereby helping to avoid varicose veins and hemorrhoids. Bran is easy to use, but does require know-how. One doesn't begin with large amounts, for there is often an initial period of intolerance, usually expressed as flatulence. I prefer beginning with a teaspoonful of bran, daily, in tablet form, or as coarse (not finely ground) bran added to cereal, applesauce, or some other vehicle of your choice. The dose is gradually increased until three objectives are reached:

1. Evacuation is easy and effortless.
2. The stool is large, soft, but well formed.
3. The stool is odorless, or nearly so. This is a token of discouragement of the unfriendly bacteria.

The physician who established the health benefits of fiber for Central Africans will not ordinarily say this when addressing a lay audience, but he adds for medical professionals a fourth objective: the stool should be lighter than water; in other words, it should float. The "sinkers," he says, are still headed for trouble.

Experience teaches us to warn newcomers to the use of bran not to stop abruptly, for the penalty will be the year's prize-winning case of abysmal constipation. I have also learned that intolerance to roughage isn't as frequent as we had supposed. For many years, it has been traditional for physicians to order a low-roughage diet for diverticulosis and diverticulitis. Realizing that a soft diet may actually be the prime cause of such disorders, medical practitioners were nonetheless loath to abandon it, for fear that the patients would have severe adverse reactions to high fiber intake. It wasn't entirely groundless an apprehension, but experience has shown that about two-thirds of those shifted to a high-fiber diet are able to tolerate and to profit by it. Allergy to wheat, though, is another matter, since bran is ordinarily of wheat origin. However, corn bran has been marketed, and may prove to be an acceptable alternative, or, in lieu of cereal bran, carrot and other vegetable fiber may be tried, though it is usually less effective than bran.

Two technical problems are created by the characteristics of bran. It is a rich source of phosphorus, and if there is anything the American diet doesn't need, it's added phosphorus. We take much protein, rich in phosphorus, from sources that do not supply balancing amounts of calcium, such as meat, fish, and fowl. Milk and its products, save cream and butter, do supply calcium with phosphorus, but we have, in the name of a misguided war against cholesterol, been discouraging the use of many dairy foods. Even if we didn't, it would still be difficult to raise calcium intake high enough to offset our high phosphorus level. The partial answer would be a calcium supplement not supplying phosphorus, which calls for the use of calcium gluconate or, preferably, calcium orotate. As the gluconate, enough is taken to yield 1 gram of calcium; as the orotate, enough to yield 300 mg., since in this form the calcium is well utilized. The increment of calcium intake serves other purposes in anticipating and preventing some of the problems of aging, in which deterioration of the skeleton in both sexes is frequent. (Many a broken bone attributed to a fall by an aged person actually precedes and causes the fall.)

What you have read explains the composition of what I have called my BAMBY plan. The acronym stands for Bran And Multiple vitamins and minerals, Brewer's yeast, and Yogurt. The calcium in the multiple mineral supplement should be augmented in the way I have described. The yogurt should be fortified with friendly bacteria, as I have indicated. Brewer's yeast (*not* torula yeast) supplies the B vitamins and other nutrients, like selenium, that are important in avoiding some of the degenerative diseases and physical and mental changes we blame on aging. One of the vitamins of the B complex is particularly important to peristalsis—the contractions of the colon that speed food residues on their way. We sometimes add additional pantothenic acid (sometimes called "pantothenol" or calcium pantothenate) to the BAMBY plan, since the amount of yeast may not be optimal.

When you consider the risks of slow transit time and the long-term penalties for it and constipation, isn't it obvious that laxatives are not the choice of the thinking person? And should you not, knowing that absence of constipation doesn't guarantee normal transit time, protect yourself against both disorders of elimination?

While the fiber of fruits and vegetables isn't as efficient as bran, it is nonetheless important in protecting us against cancer, in which action carotene (the vegetable precursor of vitamin A) is also important. My hidden motive in telling you that derives from long experience. I don't want you to add bran to an inferior diet, low in vegetables and fruits, and feel virtuous. You'll be diluting the protection.

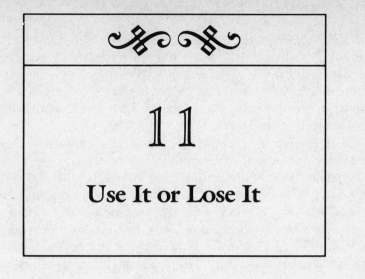

11

Use It or Lose It

When Yankee Stadium was rebuilt, it wasn't by choice that the architects installed seven thousand fewer seats than originally planned. The decision was made by the need of baseball fans for wider seats to accommodate wider bottoms. To that acknowledgment of the toll of the sedentary life, add this one: a physician, writing in the *Journal of the American Medical Association,* remarks: "In reviewing the changes commonly attributed to the process of aging, I was struck by the coincidence of many of these with changes that accompany physical inactivity."

These considerations inspire this appraisal of exercise as an anti-aging practice. It doesn't necessarily reflect my personal philosophy, for whenever I feel like exercising, I lie down until the disturbance passes away. I certainly have no quarrel with those devoted to it; only with those who, like dancers, insist that to be normal you must enjoy it. They forget individual differences, which operate in tolerance for exercise as they do in food tolerances. How many times do we see the Churchills—those whose principal exercise is lifting a cigar and a glass of brandy—survive with unimpaired function to a ripe old age? And how many times do we hear of someone, obviously not gaited for exercise, whose dividend from it was a heart attack?

The prelude to exercise, obviously, is a competent complete physical examination, including a stress tolerance test. There is a possible flaw in that test, though, for an electrocardiogram (EKG) appraises heart performance, and that fleeting electronic inspection is what? A twenty-second look at the electrical characteristics of the heart? Have we not all heard of a patient who has been assured, on the basis of an EKG, with or without stress, that his heart is normal, who nonetheless dies with a cardiac attack, minutes, hours, or days later?

Obviously aware of the limitations of an EKG of the type obtained in the medical office, physicians have resorted to a portable machine that one wears for a full twenty-four hours. This is better but not perfect, for the electronic information is compressed into but two channels, as against the many used with the nonportable machines; and disturbances again may be missed. Recently, a portable unit that is actually a computer has been developed. You wear this for twenty-four hours, after which the physician plugs it into a larger computer, which extracts from the little unit thousands of readings, actually identifying, counting, and totaling the count of deviations from the normal.

To make this type of heart examination even more efficient, there is nuclear cardiography. Radioactive material with a short half-life, thereby presenting no risk of excessive radiation, is injected intravenously. A special camera photographs the journey of the agent through the body. The pictures are computer-enhanced, and actually yield a picture in color of the beating heart. Moreover, the colors are indicative of the efficiency of the pumping of the organ, and thereby give the cardiologist a basis for estimating the degree, if any, to which the circulation through the coronaries (the vessels supplying the heart muscle with blood) are compromised. If you are an elder, the investment in these precautions is mandatory, if you want to be safe in beginning or in continuing exercise. If you are young or aging, it's advisable.

That leaves open the question whether or not exercise is a help in resisting aging. Certainly, there are athletes who die young, and "old-timers' day" at the ballpark reminds you that stalwart young athletes can in a few decades turn into toothless wrecks. I can't resist telling you that athletes don't necessarily eat properly. I was the nutritionist for the Kansas City Athletics the year they finished at the bottom of the league, and from firsthand observation I can report the tonnage of Cokes, candy, and ice cream they consumed. Part of the accelerated aging we see in these athletes, then, serves to remind us that exercise isn't an antidote for a poor diet; if anything, it will magnify its harmful effects, for stress increases nutritional needs. However, and this is the point toward which I aim this discussion, there is a remarkable overlapping of the changes attributed to aging and those which come to the sedentary. Considering what we have learned about the lethal qualities of bed rest, that statement should come as no surprise.

When we discuss the sedentary life, and compare it with bed rest, you should remember that merely staying in bed long enough can make a healthy person ill. Oxygen consumption by the body drops, and in that we are dimming the spark of life. It even goes down when a patient is confined to a chair. Conversely, exercise in bed has increased oxygen consumption. As you might expect, athletes in peak condition have very high levels of oxygen consumption.

There are two primary keys to our ability to put oxygen to work. There are nutritional factors in the use and the conservation of oxygen, and there are the physical factors, the heart and the vascular system. As we grow older, the output of the heart goes down, with each beat moving a smaller volume of blood and thereby a reduced supply of oxygen. When we age, the resting heart rate doesn't ordinarily change, but the maximum rate goes down. Exactly the same changes are produced by bed rest: the volume of blood pumped with each heart stroke dropping about 30 percent. These changes resulting from inactivity are indistinguishable from those which have been blamed on aging. There *is* one difference. The undesirable effects of bed rest or the sedentary life in the young can be reversed by exercise and improved diet. Not exactly so with the elderly: for them, exercise won't do it, but improved nutrition *will,* and that is a golden and neglected opportunity for the aged.

Blood pressure reacts to the same forces. The systolic pressure (the first figure your doctor quotes, which is the pressure when the heart is pumping) increases with age, but even in elderly people, it falls with a program of exercise. For some, it can be reduced even more by higher potassium* and lower sodium intake. This all translates simply: the steady rise in systolic blood pressure, year by year, may be average but isn't normal, and in many cases may be due to diet and to sedentary life.

There are many elderly people whose sense of balance is disturbed. In some of these cases, the cause is called "postural hypotension," meaning that the blood pressure drops significantly when they lie down or are placed on a tilt table; but exactly the same reaction occurs in individuals who are physically inactive. Both age and inactivity diminish the red blood cell mass. Both age and inactivity create a tendency to blood clots and the complications that accompany them. Both the inactive and the aging tend to higher levels of blood cholesterol and triglycerides. The sedentary person shares with old people a loss of lean (protein) body mass. Indeed, the negative protein balance created by bed rest can be so great that the diet, however high in protein, can't compensate for it. The same phenomenon appears with calcium metabolism, for the mineral departs from the bones in the aged, with a resulting tendency to fractures (blamed on falls that actually were caused by a preceding fracture). In the same way, bed rest causes a loss of calcium. Both these phenomena were part of the problems of weightlessness in space, the astronauts going into both negative protein balance and calcium balance. In fact, the effects are severe enough to prohibit space flights of more than nine months, unless preventive measures can be found. The point to all this is the same: lack of exercise creates problems indistinguishable from those blamed on aging.

Without boring you with anatomical and biochemical details, let me summarize by noting that the changes attributed to aging are duplicated by the changes clearly caused by lack of exercise, and among these, there is loss of neurotransmitters from the lower brain and spinal cord, lowering of male hormone level, fall in body temperature, disturbances of the central nervous system, in the pattern of sleep, in sense organ functions, such as taste, and in the

Not by use of supplements; use food sources.

immune system. Pertinent is the remark by a physician whose right leg was placed in a cast for six weeks. When it was removed, he was shocked to find the leg looking like that of a person forty years older than he. We can conclude that exercise won't obstruct the sand in the hourglass of time, but inactivity may make it flow faster. We can equate exercise with good nutrition in helping us to approach our potential for longevity, with vigor in the added years.

Assuming that you've been cleared medically, and not with a treadmill test preceded and followed by the usual type of EKG, what exercise do you choose, within the limitations of your cardio-vascular capacity? The list of (mostly) minor but painful disorders that joggers suffer would not make jogging ideal. Tennis and the more demanding sports are fine if you're fit, but don't forget that one of our top-seeded players, Arthur Ashe, had to retire, young as he was, because of a heart attack. The Greeks had a word for it, which is useful for both exercise and nutrition: moderation. If I must vote for ideal exercises, not based on personal preference but on potential benefit and reasonable safety, I'd vote for swimming and for the use of a small trampoline, now available in sizes appropriate for the home or office. Both are to be explored in moderation. I have been known to observe that I have derived too much exercise as a pallbearer for friends on the low-cholesterol diet who overexercised.

Orthodox dietitians and nutritionists will tell you that there is no special diet and there are no particular nutrients that improve athletic performance. They should have read the reports from the physical fitness department of the University of Illinois, which for years exhaustively studied the combined effects of nutritional sup-plementing and exercise. The results were startling, for the subjects, including both athletes and nonathletes in poor physical condition, responded dramatically to supplements of a concentrate of wheat germ oil, coupled with a regimen of exercise gaited to individual needs and tolerances. The net effect, to paraphrase their technical language, was to turn the physiological clock back for the sedentary subjects, with fifty-year-olds performing like forty-year-olds. That is a remarkable result, considering that the performance pathway begins to tilt downward before puberty. Ten-year-olds will emerge from all-out running less exhausted than fourteen-year-olds.

The supplement used in the University of Illinois studies is octocosanol, which is a nutrient important to muscle performance.

It is normal to the diet, being supplied by the germ of whole grains and by green leafy vegetables. Millions of capsules of octocosanol have been used regularly by athletes, and it is time the inactive caught up with its usefulness when coupled with planned exercise. The health food stores stock it, a 2-mg. potency the usual recommended intake. Synthetic octocosanol has been marketed, but I prefer the type derived from and accompanied by wheat germ oil, which supplies other nutrients of the same chemical family—long-chain, waxy alcohols—which also have physiological activity and which are not present in the synthetic concentrates. For the technically minded, these include hexacosanol, tetracosanol, and triacontinol. All these factors have beneficial effects other than their stimulation of muscle function, some of which will be discussed later in the context of degeneration of the brain.

To this point, the discussion has been aimed at both sexes, but women have some problems (other than men) that must pointedly be addressed. As a woman, when you wish to capitalize on exercise as an anti-aging force, you have a problem that is uniquely feminine. If you overdo it, you may create hormone disturbances that can stop the menstruals. It is a temporary effect, but obviously calls for temperance in exercise.

With exercise clearly an anti-aging activity for younger women, it has a special importance for those approaching the menopausal years. As you must know, this is a decade in which changes in glandular function may play havoc with the skeleton, with loss of calcium that can be both painful and disfiguring. Orthodox medical management of the problem will have you gulping pills of estrogen and fluoride, as undesirable a therapy as any of those which give nutritionists nightmares. In addition to the possible dangers of the drug treatment, it is a striking example of crisis medicine used where prevention could have been applied. The woman whose lifetime intake of calcium is generous, say 1,500 mg. daily, is much less likely to develop osteoporosis. There are also dividends in protecting the skeleton by appropriate exercise. A vertical impact on the skeleton generates electrical activity that tends to attract calcium to the bones. This phenomenon helps to protect the supporting structures of the teeth, and lack of the vertical impact of chewing creates some of the disorders that keep periodontists busy. This explains the loss of bone in those who must wear dentures, and in those who lose teeth and do not replace them. It also explains why skipping rope, which obviously represents a vertical impact upon the skeleton, is an excellent exercise for women at any age, and particularly when approaching the menopause. If you are not a devotee of rope-skipping, the small trampoline is a moderately effective substitute.

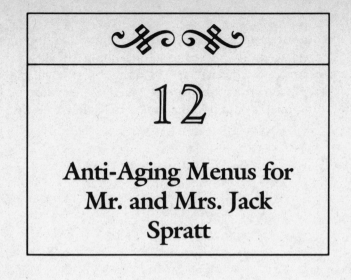

12

Anti-Aging Menus for Mr. and Mrs. Jack Spratt

On what basis do Americans select their foods and beverages? I once tried the experiment of stopping supermarket shoppers as they retrieved their purchases from the carts and loaded them into their cars, and asked on what criteria their selections were based. Only infrequently did their answers have anything to do with maintenance of health, recovery from illness, or delaying of aging.

Impulse was a strong influence. So were sales, seasonal availability, and coupon discounts. Sometimes the attraction was a reusable container. Habit played a dominant role, voiced in "We always have chicken on Wednesday." Family tradition, often reflecting ethnic customs, strongly operated: "We Italians like pasta." Or "My mother always bought/made that." Religion dictated many choices, ranging from fish on Friday to the choice of the constituents of an all-dairy meal. Budgets, of course, made some choices and some rejections mandatory: "I can't afford tuna fish; that's why I bought macaroni and cheese." Or "I don't like hamburger, but who can buy decent steaks at today's prices?"

Restrictions on the diet for medical reasons are frequent. Allergies prohibit the purchase of many common foods and dictate selection of alternatives. So do medically prescribed diets for treatment of ulcer, irritable bowel, or cardiovascular diseases.

Rare, obviously, is the shopper whose response is "I bought that because it's important to a balanced diet." Balanced for whom? is the question we must now address as we explore the individual differences that reflect the "me" in menus and the "I" in diet for prolonging the prime of life.

Least popular with my lecture, broadcast, and classroom audiences is a discussion of individual differences in nutritional requirements. The public prefers pat answers, wants dogma rather than discussion, finding rather than seeking. Not for nothing did John Dewey remark that Americans would rather know than think, for certainty is free from anxiety. Yet any nutritionist worthy of the title knows that two men of the same height and weight, eating the same amounts of the same foods, may produce energy by totally different biochemical pathways, and one may produce more fat and less energy than the other. How many times have *you* perhaps complained that others may eat desserts without weight gain, while you put on pounds if you smell a cake baking? I'll discuss that phenomenon in this chapter, for not only does this biochemical idiosyncrasy exist, but for displaying it, many innocents have been accused of cheating on their reducing diets.

Consider some of the anatomical and biochemical differences that make each of us unique. We are all normally born with beta cells on the pancreas, which produce insulin. Some of us have 250,000 such cells, and some have over two million. Insulin being required for utilization and recycling of starches and sugars, consider the implications of this difference in carbohydrate tolerance. This could mean greater susceptibility to diabetes or to low blood sugar if the carbohydrate load overtaxes the limited capacity of the pancreas to deal with it, or drives it beyond its normal limits. And how could there then be a single ideal amount of sugar and starch to be specified as the recommended dietary allowance?

We all vitally need intake of vitamin B complex and protein. But the breakdown of estrogen (female hormone) by the liver is, like so many other processes in the body, dependent on adequate intake of these dietary factors. Women, though, differ in estrogen production by a factor of at least five, and controlling the activity of the hormone is essential to reduce the risk of estrogen-dependent cancer of the breast and uterus, to help avoid uterine fibroid tumors, and to minimize the symptoms many women suffer in the menstrual. The high-estrogen lady will have a high requirement for these vitamins and amino acids.

In my discussion of exercise, you read that bed rest, like the weightlessness experienced by the astronauts, can cause losses of skeletal calcium. Few noticed, though, that one astronaut in three of those studied in weightlessness escaped this penalty for lack of gravity, suffering no changes in bone density. His immunity freed him from the elevated calcium requirement needed by his companions.

Animals with an inborn deficiency in cytochrome P-450 or a lack of brown fat will grow obese on a high-carbohydrate diet, which has no such effect on animals well supplied with the enzyme. Moreover, the deficit in the enzyme becomes more severe as the animals age. One is reminded of the obese who complain that as the years accumulate, weight loss becomes increasingly difficult to achieve. Such individuals can't tolerate what is erroneously described as the "normal" carbohydrate intake. The rest of us, consuming as much as a ton of food per year, find that the wisdom of the body maintains our weight at a fairly stable level, varying but two or three pounds.

The heart may pump as little as four liters of blood per minute, or up to ten. Consider the differences in oxygen supplies to the tissues, and the differing needs for iron and protein for hemoglobin, and in vitamin-mineral-protein supplies for blood enzymes.

The amount of sugar you use to make a beverage taste sweet may be genetically determined. A 5 percent solution of sugar in water tastes sweet to a majority, but there are those who will not detect sweetness until nearly *thirteen* teaspoonfuls of sugar have been added. In the backgrounds of children with this characteristic, there is often a history of diabetes in the family, and we can't decide whether this taste aberration induces consumption of more sugar and thereby fans the flame of a latent diabetes. The alternative, of course, would be that the tendency to the disease creates the inability to detect sweetness until it is concentrated to the point where the average individual would find it sickening. Here you see the influence of an individual difference on food selections and ultimately on health and longevity.

I mentioned earlier that Dr. Linus Pauling estimates that individual differences dictate a range of vitamin C requirement from as little as 250 mg. daily to 2,500 mg. We see exactly the same range in animals like guinea pigs, which require an external source of the vitamin, as man does. There are guinea pigs that remain free of scurvy on one-fifth the amount the species ordinarily requires, and there are those whose need is twenty times greater. This biochemical individuality means that I may have second-grade health on a vitamin C intake that is your requirement for optimal well-being.

Those who have seen the human wrecks rescued from the concentration camps of World War II need no persuasion to recognize that generalizations about dietary adequacy or inadequacy are simply impermissible. Some of the prisoners had beriberi, some had scurvy, some had pellagra; all were skin and bones, but there were those who were remarkably free of dietary deficiency diseases.

What you have already read must have persuaded you not to expect a set of menus for those who want to slow down or reverse aging, for you, like one of Shakespeare's protagonists, display infinite variety. We can and must build a dietetic structure of whatever generalizations are permissible, and follow that with guidelines from that point to shape your nutrition to meet your individual requirements and tolerances. There *are* nutritional tests that can tell us a great deal about your vitamin, mineral, and protein needs, but we don't have them for all the nutrients, and frequently, the information they yield is but a partial guide. We can roughly generalize about requirements for protein foods, but must cope not only with great variations in need but those in tolerances, such as the limitations created by the less efficient protein utilization (and excessive excretion of nitrogen) in the aged.

After a fatty meal, the blood of a youngster remains milky for a short time. When the milkiness disappears, the body has utilized that supply of fat. The clearing period is very much longer for the aging and the aged. This, like the failing utilization of protein, calls for special measures to improve both the absorption and the utilization of fats. Another variable is tolerance for vegetable oils as compared with tolerance for animal fats. There are remedial procedures in nutrition for this problem, too.

From the discussion of the pancreatic beta cells, cytochrome P-450, and brown fat, you already know that it isn't possible to generalize about the starch-sugar needs. There are those who thrive on a high intake of complex carbohydrate, meaning starches rather than sugars; and there are those who will never be truly well until they are placed on a low-carbohydrate diet. "Low-carbohydrate," contrary to popular medical and lay opinion, does not necessarily mean high-protein, high-fat. You yourself have noticed that a steak sticks to your ribs; an equal number of calories from bread or cereal don't. In fact, you've complained about the lack of the stick-to-the-ribs quality of low-protein, low-fat meals, remarking that an hour after such a meal in a Chinese restaurant, you're hungry again. This is a way of acknowledging that protein and fat, for most people, have great satiety effects. That is why some people, those who can resist anything but temptation, will lose weight effectively only on low-carbohydrate diets. Others do as well on the conventional 1,200-calorie menus. For some, weight loss is elusive unless the 1,200-calorie diet contains the amount of protein normal to a diet twice as high in calories. That, incidentally, is the secret of the so-called Scarsdale diet.

I obviously can't tell you the whole story of individual differences in man's biochemistry and nutritional needs and tolerances, for whole textbooks have been devoted to that subject. I've accomplished my objective if you are now aware that you and I are unique events in the biochemical universe, and that no one has the right to generalize about our needs in food.

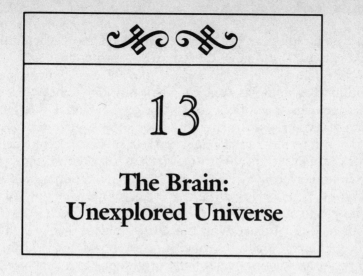

13

The Brain:
Unexplored Universe

Though space is often called "the last frontier," it is man's brain which is driven to explore it and man's mind which must understand it. Paradoxically, we know more about space and celestial bodies than we do about our brains. Although Alexander Pope suggested that the proper study for man is man, we have long ignored the near-at-hand and have pondered instead the remote and the unapproachable.

Whenever I read a vitamin and health food catalogue, I am troubled by some of the dogmatic statements concerning nutrients essential to brain function, such as "Tryptophane improves depression" and "Lecithin helps memory." These confident claims remind me of the remark made by a neurologist who was asked what the future held for a brain-damaged patient whose electroencephalogram was blank where important electrical activity in the brain should have been displayed. "Absence of the alpha wave," he said, "has no meaning we can interpret. We don't know where thinking takes place." The vitamin catalogues do, apparently.

Beginning with that negative note, I am about to tell you within what limits we are able to apply nutrition to help the brain to manage both its emotions and its thinking. I wanted, though, to be sure that you know the sparsity of our knowledge of the chemistry of brain function. Let's begin with the history of a lecture delivered by a distinguished psychiatrist more than half a century ago. He was attempting to convince his peers that the mind can make the body sick or well. His reward was the jeering of his fellow psychiatrists, who proposed that he join the Christian Science church, and his widow, long a listener to my broadcasts, told me that he died with a broken heart, though his concept of psychosomatic medicine was, in the usual lagging way of the profession, later embraced. The histories I am about to relate are a tribute to the foresight of Dr. Smith Ely Jelliffe. They also teach a profound (and frequently overlooked) lesson to you who would like to remain young, productive, and healthy into the senior years.

The first history is that of a terminal cancer patient who pleaded with his physician for treatment with a "quack" remedy, then called "Krebiozen." The doctor, fully aware that the patient would not survive long, obtained this unlicensed medication and was amazed when the cancer, of a type visible to the eye, shrank to half its former size as Krebiozen was administered, with the patient clinically obviously much improved. At that point, the American Medical Association and the Food and Drug Administration issued simultaneous bulletins, warning the public and the profession that Krebiozen was completely useless. The cancer returned to its original size, though the doctor continued the injections, and the patient was again terminal. Now the physician told the sufferer that he had obtained a special batch of Krebiozen which, contrary to the official position, was extremely potent as an anticancer drug. The doctor proceeded to give repeated injections of distilled water, and the cancer again shrank, and the patient clinically improved again. Then came a fresh blast from the medical society and the government agency, saying that analysis of Krebiozen showed it to be nothing more than a simple, totally inactive protein material. The patient died one week later.

The second history is that of a little boy, terminal with a type of brain cancer that is resistant to chemotherapy and irradiation, occupying so large an area of the brain as to be inoperable. His desperate family took him to a professional team, husband and wife, who had success in using mental imagery in the treatment of certain types of cancer. The child was taught to visualize the cancer cells as the "bad guys" and the immune cells, normal to the body as part of its defense mechanism, as the "good guys." The child, with the vivid imagination of a small boy, followed the instructions, deviating only by visualizing the "good guys" as little doctors, armed with lances and attacking the "bad guys." Though he had been pronounced terminal, the child improved steadily, until there came the day when he told his father: "I can't see the bad guys anymore. All I see is a white line." His father urged him to try harder, but when the child persisted in his statements, the father took him to a cancer hospital for a brain scan. It revealed a thin line of scar tissue as the only residue of what had been a rapidly growing and lethal cancer.

These histories did not originate with a supermarket tabloid. They came from the published observations of competent physicians, writing in reputable medical journals. They asseverate the link between the brain and the immune system, a tie so intimate that one must be persuaded that passive patients die faster with cancer because the conversation between the brain and the defense system has been interrupted, garbled, or distorted because there is a death wish at the brain (or even the cellular) level. These aspects of the mysteries of man's brain will not be understood by assays of brain enzymes or by scans of the glucose fires within our skulls. Though there is a whole textbook on the detailed anatomy of the brain, examined microscopically thin slice by slice, that will not unlock the mysteries either. This, though, we are beginning to understand: when the relationship between your brain and your immune system is disturbed, when your mind is no longer your friend, I am convinced that taking nutrients that stimulate the brain or immune system becomes an exercise in futility. This is not to diminish the importance to cerebral metabolism and to the immune system of nutrition aimed at maximum efficiency. Rather, it is to emphasize that your attitudes and emotions are, in a very real sense, part of the complex chains of reactions in which nutrients are also indispensable links.

Dr. Bernard Rimland has aptly called the brain the "soggy computer." In it, the equivalent of the wires in an electronic computer are liquids containing chemicals called neurotransmitters.

There are at least twenty-five of these compounds at work in the brain, some of which excite nerve cells and some of which quiet them. One of these is serotonin, which is usually a calming neurotransmitter. With a deficit in it, just by way of illustrating the mysteries we dimly perceive, you may become a victim of obsessive-compulsive behavior, which may disappear if we give you the amino acid that encourages production of serotonin. On the other hand, if you are a victim of compulsions and also have a history of violent behavior, the "quieting" neurotransmitter may make you aggressive and asocial. By way of underscoring our difficulties in understanding these contradictory effects, if you elevate your serotonin level too much for you, though not necessarily for the next person, the calming neurotransmitter may reverse its role and become an overstimulator. Still more contradictions fascinate (though they currently baffle) us. In the brains of psychopathic killers, there is a deficiency in serotonin. One study revealed a low serotonin level in a markedly depressed survivor in a family in which there had been a number of suicides. So did an examination of the brain of a member of the family who had recently killed himself. Raising the serotonin activity in the survivor eliminated the self-destructiveness.

Given the precursor of the body's manufacture of serotonin, which is the protein (amino acid) tryptophane, some people enjoy reduced sleep latency, a significant shortening of the interval between closing one's eyes and actually falling asleep; others enjoy no such dividend. The same differences appear in reactions to ion generators, which produce negative ions and raise serotonin levels, promoting heightened well-being and deeper sleep. For *some* people. Isn't this also true of the time-honored sleep-producing device, a glass of hot milk before retiring? Milk supplies tryptophane and calcium, quieting nutrients. For *some* people.

While this discussion may seem remote from the subject of this book, be patient with me. I have a point to make which will be very important in your effort to remain young and productive through the later years.

It is important to understand that a deficit in serotonin (or, for that matter, an oversupply) may be biogenic or sociogenic. In other words, it may originate with your life situation or with a vagary of body chemistry, or with an inadequate diet, or with a combination of these. Whether your depression is caused by catastrophic events or disturbed chemistry, in that order, or begins with disturbed chemistry, which then causes depression, the cycle must be broken if you are to recover; and it doesn't matter at what point you break out of the circle. You may choose to unburden yourself by conversation with a psychiatrist, or you may visit an orthomolecular practitioner for appropriate nutritional therapy, or, better yet, you do both, but the end result of successful therapy will be the same. If your depression leaves, it will be because you have raised brain serotonin activity. This, among many other possible conclusions, tells you that there is no valid reason for the hostility of the conventional psychiatrist toward the orthomolecular psychiatrist. They are both treating the same elephant, though from different directions. The conventional practitioner is changing brain chemistry with conversation, calmative drugs, or shock therapy. The orthomolecular practitioner is doing it with nutrients normal to the body.

With that theoretical explanation behind us, oversimplified though it is, the moral should be plain. The depression that is almost indigenous to old age may be avoided with adequate intake of tryptophane, vitamin B_6, and niacinamide. You must not forget though, that any computer can be overridden, and that your attitude toward old age is as critical a "nutrient" as any derived from food.

The same interaction of the biogenic and the sociogenic occurs with the neurotransmitter involved in short-term memory. This, acetylcholine, is created in your body from pantothenic acid, choline, and manganese. When your acetylcholine brain level falls, you may find yourself infuriatingly unable to remember events of yesterday, but absolutely sure of occurrences decades ago. This once was explained by conceiving of the brain as a blank slate that, with the accumulated memories of the years, ultimately becomes filled with data, leaving no room to inscribe recent memories. That, though, is like blaming arthritis on old age, inviting the logical response: what about the aged who are not arthritic? Similarly, there are the elderly who have excellent memories, both short-term and long-term. (Case in point: I am writing this entire chapter without reference to a single text or note, and today is my seventy-second birthday.) In the course of experiments in raising brain levels of acetylcholine, researchers encountered improvements in short-term memory. However, the same result came with vitamin B_6, which is not involved in acetylcholine synthesis, which rests on pantothenic acid (another B vitamin), plus choline and manganese. This led to direct use of choline, as a step nearer to encouragement of acetylcholine synthesis in the brain. Fascinatingly, not only did this improve short-term memory in the aged and senile, though it is no panacea; it also helped short-term memory in normal young individuals. And, by way of complicating matters still more, vitamin B_6 proved helpful in remembering dreams, a faculty that obviously involves short-term memory. My educated hunch: we are in the kindergarten stage of this research, and will graduate to advanced classes when we devote more study to the modulators, which determine the action of the neurotransmitters.

Still another neurotransmitter, actually a group of them, the catecholamines, were also studied. The dietary precursor for these is tyrosine, an amino acid that the body manufactures from another amino acid, phenylalanine. It was logical to pursue this chemistry for depressed patients, since the catecholamines are stimulating neurotransmitters. So it was discovered that depression may have more than one biochemical origin, for some patients were helped with phenylalanine who did not respond to tryptophane.

Another amino acid was long ago found to benefit brain function. This was glutamic acid. The discovery derived originally from studies of the improvement in mental function of rats dosed with the protein. The animals had to learn to step on switches to open the door to the food box. The sequence in which the switches had to be energized was random, requiring an astonishingly high level of intelligence for the animals to discover (and remember) the correct sequence. One of these rats learned a five-switch sequence, a task that might very well have defeated a child (and some adults). Later, it was realized that glutamic acid does not efficiently penetrate the barrier between the blood circulation and the brain, a mechanism that is most selective about the substances (and amounts of them) it will permit to pass. This suggested a change to the administration of a factor that the brain converts into glutamic acid: L glutamine, which readily passes the barrier. A marked stimulant to the brain and the central nervous system, L glutamine has also been found very helpful in eliminating the craving for alcohol in confirmed alcoholics. It has stimulated brain function, both in the normal and in the retarded, though, paradoxically, most of the nutritional research has been confined to Downs syndrome and other types of mental retardation, and for the most part in children. I don't understand the assumption that improved nutrition yields dividends only to slow minds, nor the underlying assumption that both the normal and the geniuses all eat diets providing optimal nutrition for the brain. As a member of Mensa, a society of those with IQs far above the average, I can tell you that many geniuses eat like idiots.

All this suggests that it is not enough to aim at nutrition good enough to retard physical aging. There is, in a real sense, brain food. Part of that is on your dining room table; some of it is in your supplements; but there are emotional and attitudinal vitamins, too. Those who remain busy and productive tend to remain capable of being busy and productive. Those who are happily occupied in pursuits that give a sense of accomplishment and recognition remain younger, both in body and mind. There is a fundamental incompatibility between old thoughts and a young body. If you have seen the kaleidoscopic swiftness of aging in a relatively young person who has had a stroke, the relationship between youth of mind and youth of body needs no further emphasis.

It was with that thought that earlier I mentioned the usefulness of vitamin C and bioflavonoids in reducing the tendency to and the toll of small strokes. Let me acquaint you with another nutrient with beneficial effects on the brain. This is octocosanol, to which I have devoted many decades of research which have been highlighted by the remarkable effects of this nutrient on some cases of severe brain damage. As part of that research, I have been responsible for administration of octocosanol to some 300 multiple sclerosis patients, whose responses indicated that octocosanol helps to restore the "insulation" (myelin sheaths), whose disappearance causes the "short-circuiting" of the nervous system, which is a component of the disease. Other responses led me to believe that this nutrient stimulates the repair of damaged brain cells (neurons), which the textbooks for decades have mistakenly declared impossible. The recoveries I have witnessed in the treatment of brain damage with octocosanol indicate that this nutrient—and it is a nutrient—may also help to protect those brain cells which are healthy. Since we routinely lose millions of cells in every organ of the body as we age, including the brain, octocosanol should be added to your list of supplements. It is best derived from concentrated wheat germ oil, in which it is accompanied by other, related compounds that are physiologically active. There are added dividends from octocosanol supplements, including an ergonomic effect, which literally means it augments energy. This explains why athletes for decades have taken octocosanol supplements to the tune of tens of millions of capsules and tablets. A supplementary intake, which seems ridiculously small but has profound effects, is 2 mg. daily. In some younger women, this nutrient has a distinct aphrodisiac effect. I have not observed this in men of any age.

RNA, a genetic-messenger compound, is depleted as the years accumulate. Vitamin B_{12} stimulates the synthesis of RNA in brain cells, which is useful in helping retention of memory, for RNA has been called a "memory molecule." Mice fed generous amounts of the physiological chemical live longer, but this may merely be the antioxidant effect of RNA. It breaks down in the body to uric acid. This is academic to most of us, but a threat to those with gout, those with elevated uric acid, and, possibly, those whose family history indicates a tendency toward gout. Your physician can, of course, test you for blood uric acid and for kidney function. If both are normal, raising your intake of RNA should be no threat. You can do so by eating sardines or by taking an RNA supplement, available in the health food stores.

Those interested in promoting acetylcholine synthesis, which is important both to the brain and the nervous system—muscle function, are sometimes puzzled by the diversity of sources of this neurotransmitter, for the list includes a proprietary drug (Deaner), lecithin, and choline itself. The drug represents a modified form of choline that more easily reaches the brain. Choline itself, in some individuals, is broken down by intestinal bacteria, causing a fish odor in the stool, in the urine, and sometimes from the individual himself. The choline in lecithin is resistant to the bacteria. Ordinary lecithin supplies much less choline than a specially processed type called "high phosphatidyl choline lecithin."

We are what we eat? True. We also think with what we eat.

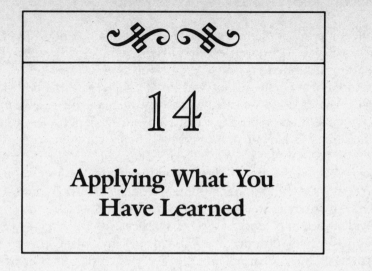

14

Applying What You Have Learned

In meeting the requirements for the Ph.D., I conducted research in which I compared the diets of a group of my radio listeners with those of a demographically equated group of nonlisteners (who had nonetheless somehow managed to survive). My hypothesis proposed that those regularly listening to broadcasts on nutrition would be better fed, and so it proved, but the superiority was not due to more intelligent selection of foods; it was achieved by the use of vitamin, mineral, and other supplements. In short, my listeners were ignoring an axiom I had repeated, over and over again: supplements are *supplements,* not licenses for poor nutrition, not substitutes for intelligent selection of foods.

You may think it's academic. What difference does it make if a vitamin reaches you via a capsule or a pill, rather than a food? The emphasis on the basic diet is necessary because there are unidentified nutrients which, being such, obviously can't be concentrated as others are in supplements. These are obtainable only from a well-selected diet. Moreover, every nutrient, almost without exception, has unique functions and can't be replaced by another. A quick example of the gaps in our knowledge will clarify the point: if we feed extra liver to animals, we vastly increase their resistance to fatigue. So much so that animals unable to swim beyond a half-hour when fed an adequate diet can extend their swimming time to over two hours when liver is added to the same diet. We can't reproduce that effect with any of the known nutrients of liver. Not with protein, not with vitamins, minerals, fats, or carbohydrates. Thus we know there is an antifatigue factor in liver, which someday may be identified and concentrated or synthesized. Until then, you who hate liver will not make up the deficit by eating other animal proteins, and no supplement—save desiccated liver itself—will supply you with this ergonomic factor. That leads us to Rule #1: Food comes first.

Rule #2: The term "well-balanced diet" is a shibboleth of dieticians and nutritionists who prefer the convenience of generalizations to the labor of wrestling with individual differences. Diseases, the genes, and stress are factors creating variations in nutritional requirements. That is why attempts to set an RDA for carbohydrate allowances are worse than useless; they're ignorant. The caveman didn't breakfast on krispy, krackly Krunchies before sallying forth to battle the saber-toothed tiger. In his environment, only fruits, shoots, tubers, and an occasional find of honey could have provided significant amounts of starches and sugars. He had plenty of energy without cereals, breads, rolls, cakes, candy, cookies, or a sugar bowl, for he early learned how to use protein and fat for enduring energy. Concentrated carbohydrates for which dietitians set an RDA were simply not available until two major discoveries were made: the invention of agriculture, first aimed at producing carbohydrates for animal feed; and the introduction of concentrated sugar. In man's long history, these innovations took place only minutes ago. Judge them by what happens when we introduce these foods today to primitives who formerly fed on protein and fat from fish. The result is that we increase their death rate from heart attacks by a factor of *ten*. A uniform RDA for carbohydrate for hundreds of millions of people whose chemistries are not uniform is worse than ignorant and stupid; it is a legal form of homicide. There are still millions of cavemen (and cavewomen) among us whose tolerance for starches and sugars is limited. Any pediatrician with experience in dietary management of childhood epilepsy knows this, for the ratio between fat and carbohydrate needed to control the convulsions will differ sharply from child to child.

Other factors create unique nutritional requirements. If you are an alcoholic, a smoker, cardiac or hypertensive, or you have arthritis, diabetes, depression, osteoporosis, or even urinary incontinence, your nutrition can and should be targeted to meet the special needs these disorders create. As an example, your tinnitus (subjective noises in your ears) isn't an ear disorder, but the result of excessively elevated blood insulin levels, making you acutely intolerant of all simple sugars, excessive intake of starch, and long intervals between meals. Even your sex can be a factor in determining the type of diet you should be eating. As a woman, you need guidance to menus low in sugar and caffeine, high in protein, and rich in the nutrients that will help you to mitigate premenstrual syndrome, regulate your cycle, and increase your resistance to cystic breast disease, uterine fibroid tumors, endometriosis, and a common type of breast cancer. If you are male and in the late forties or early fifties, it would be helpful to you to arrange both your diet and supplements to minimize the effects of benign enlargement of the prostate, which tortures many older men.

The medications you may be taking modify your nutritional needs, too. The birth control pill critically raises the requirements for vitamin A, vitamin C, and the vitamin B complex. The diuretics prescribed for hypertensive patients can cause dehydration, lowering blood volume and making you more vulnerable to paralysis from a stroke. It is the task of the nutritionist to plan your scheme of things dietetic to minimize the danger, though I must add that the hypertension medications are themselves dangerous, and we are often successful in lowering blood pressure nutritionally, without drugs.

What you are about to read summarizes the ways in which the nutritionist can mold your diet and your supplements to meet your unique requirements. As you read this, keep in mind that many of the "truths" everyone accepts about nutrition are fairy tales, though accepted as articles of faith by incautious dietitians and physicians. For example: you'd expect a fast to cause faster weight loss than a

1,000-calorie diet. Not so. You wouldn't expect the frequency of meals to make any difference in your response to a diet. It does. More frequent, small meals, replacing the same amount of food usually taken in three meals, will be more efficient in controlling weight, in inducing weight loss, in stabilizing carbohydrate metabolism, and in normalizing such blood lipids as cholesterol and triglycerides. Observations like these explain why the study of you as an individual is a sine qua non in determining what (and when) you should be eating.

Striking differences appear in carbohydrate metabolism, and are revealed by a glucose tolerance test, which is the cornerstone of medical appraisal of your reaction to starches and sugars. In a recent study by United States Department of Agriculture researchers at the Carbohydrate Laboratory of the agency, 20 percent of the healthy males tested had abnormal reactions to quantities of sugar "normally" consumed by the average American. Sugar, of course, is but one of the carbohydrates you consume, though it is the one you most signally abuse, the average intake being, preposterously, a teaspoonful every thirty-five minutes, twenty-four hours daily. Sugar appears in the diet not only as table sugar and in thousands of processed foods, but also in fruits, some vegetables, honey, molasses, corn syrup, and as a byproduct of metabolism of such carbohydrates as sorbitol and mannitol—with which some "dietetic" and "sugar-free" chewing gums and confections are laden. Their calorie value is the same as that of sucrose (white sugar.) The complex starches, such as the whole grains, are not a stress upon the body, as sugars are, because, among other reasons, they are digested and utilized more slowly. There is an obvious price for "quick energy." It is called "fatigue"!

Determining your optimal carbohydrate intake will sound like a complex procedure. Actually, it isn't, but it is best supervised by a nutritionist, for healthy people and, mandatorily so, for those who are obese, diabetic, or hypoglycemic.

TESTING FOR OPTIMAL CARBOHYDRATE INTAKE

The first step is the glucose tolerance test, which measures the blood sugar levels at intervals, after a dose of sugar. This will identify not only the diabetic and those with low blood sugar, but also those who should restrict or eliminate, so far as possible, any intake of sugar. It also will help in determining the intake of starches appropriate for the individual. Since the test itself may cause malaise, those who have symptoms after it must wait until the next day, at least, to begin their test of carbohydrate depletion, which is the next step. This may be attempted at two levels of carbohydrate intake: zero, and 60 grams. The choice is dictated by the person's reactions to the glucose tolerance test. Some people are still not feeling well three or four days after the dose of sugar; most recover by the next day. Similarly, some feel very well on zero carbohydrate, and, indeed, some insulin-dependent diabetics find, to their amazement, that such a diet allows them, under careful, competent medical supervision, to reduce and in some cases even to eliminate their insulin injections or hypoglycemic oral drugs. Others, diabetic or not, may find zero carbohydrate to be debilitating, as the body shifts its energy source from starches and sugars to fat, so much so that they are unable to struggle through the first few days of carbohydrate deprivation, to reach the next plateau, where they begin to feel better, sometimes, than ever they have before.

The glucose tolerance test will also identify those who are not diabetic, but are en route to the disorder; and that applies to low blood sugar, too. There are some common errors to be avoided by the physician administering and interpreting the test. It should not be interpreted by the numbers, meaning the serial glucose levels alone, for any symptoms you develop in response to a dose of sugar are pertinent. It should not be a two- or three-hour test, though that mistake is often made, for the disturbances in carbohydrate tolerance may not appear until the fifth or sixth hour. Some of them may be so fleeting that it may be necessary to sample blood levels of glucose at five-minute intervals, for they otherwise may be missed. Finally, the test should never be performed without an attendant in the room, for on occasion, supposedly normal patients have reacted to a dose of sugar with convulsions in the last two hours of the test.

After the glucose tolerance test, some subjects, by way of demonstrating individual differences, have symptoms of weakness, lassitude, and headaches. If so, this calls for a day's delay in starting the test for carbohydrate deprivation. On the second day, a menu plan eliminating all starches and sugars is followed. This allows all meats save organ meats, salami, bologna, and meat dishes with fillers (bread, bread crumbs, Hamburger Helper, etc.). Eggs are not restricted. It should be emphasized that the fallacies in the cholesterol theory often are revealed here, for blood cholesterol usually *drops* during the carbohydrate-deprivation week, despite a high intake of foods containing it. So do triglyceride levels. All kinds of fowl, without stuffing, are permitted. Diet gelatin desserts are allowed, if the carbohydrate content is "zero" or "trace," though the artificial colors and flavors in these products are no boon. Regular Jell-O contains them, as well as 85 percent sugar, which bars this form of the dessert. Artificial sweeteners are allowed, but those in the granulated form, which usually contain carbohydrates, are limited to two packets daily. All seasonings are permitted, save ketchup and other tomato products or seasonings with a high sugar content.

The hard cheeses and the semisoft are permissible, but cheese spreads, diet cheeses, and cheese "foods" often contain carbohydrate and are off-limits. Cottage, pot, farmer, hoop, and ricotta are the fresh cheeses permitted. Avoid the diet cheeses in this fresh category. Tofu is permissible. Salads should be based on leafy greens, plus celery, cucumber, radish, bean sprouts, and peppers. Tomatoes, carrots, and onions are taboo. Oil, vinegar, and all spices that are free of sugar and starch are permitted, as well as the usual salad garnishes, such as anchovies, nitrite-free bacon (available in most health food stores), eggs, and grated cheese. Labels of prepared salad dressings should be carefully read, for many contain sugar. The cold-pressed oils are preferable, and available in the health food stores. These include sesame, soy, safflower, and sunflower seed oil. In any case, wherever purchased, the oil should not contain BHA or BHT. This does not mean that butter and other saturated fats and mayonnaise are forbidden, but quantities should be moderate. Beverages include spring water, Perrier, Mountain Valley, and Vichy, though tap water and club soda are allowed. Sugar-free herbal teas, free of caffeine, are preferred to coffee and ordinary tea, though decaffeinated coffee is permitted. So are clear broth and dehydrated bouillons, though some of these contain as much as 3 grams of carbohydrate—sugar or starch, or both—and you are limited to one serving daily. Alcohol is verboten during this period.

With this plan, you might breakfast on eggs in any form, made without milk, plus bacon, ham, smoked fish, or cheese, with a beverage from the approved list. For lunch you have your choice of a protein food, which might be fowl, meat, seafood, cheese, or eggs, or a palatable combination of these, with a small tossed green salad, plus an approved dressing and beverage. Dinner might open with a sauceless seafood cocktail or smoked fish, followed by broiled or sautéed fish or meat in butter, with another green salad with approved dressing and beverage. It must be emphasized that during this week of carbohydrate wipe-out, the smallest cheating will distort the results. That means that even a gumdrop or a piece of chewing gum will negate the entire test. There will be a group for whom this type of zero carbohydrate intake will be a rewarding, lifetime practice. A much larger group, though, will find it a guide to a lifetime diet in which starches will be a necessary part, though in quantities much smaller, probably, than they had formerly consumed.

When you give your report on your week's experience with the diet, your physician will perform a ketone test, which measures your efficiency in using fat, rather than carbohydrate, as a primary fuel. Other laboratory tests, including blood fats, will be performed. The findings will then be applied in shaping your permanent diet. For example, the nutritionist may instruct you to add a nutritious cereal to your breakfast, and a slice of whole wheat bread to lunch and/or dinner. Each increment in carbohydrate intake will be evaluated, until the laboratory reports and your personal reactions indicate that you have reached your optimal carbohydrate intake. Right now that is dictated by your craving for cookies, bread, cake, candy, or soda pop. You will find the scientific approach much more rewarding as a guide to lifetime nutrition for optimal health and resistance to disease.

While the procedure I've just described is that of a number of medical nutritionists in establishing optimal carbohydrate intake, I myself have used another approach. It is intended to avoid ketosis and the symptoms it causes in some people. I reduce the carbohydrate to 60 grams daily, a level well tolerated by the large majority of people, though it is far below the starch-sugar intake in the average American diet. (This procedure is *not* for diabetics.) I then suggest cautious experiments, both in raising and lowering that intake. This can be a critical determination, for some subjects. I have told the story of a student of mine, now a nutrition educator, who was a severe hypoglycemic, and rescued himself with my diet for low blood sugar, which initially sets carbohydrate intake at 60 grams daily, from starches, without sugar. After twenty years on the diet, during which he rescued himself also from what had been misdiagnosed as mental retardation, my student reported that he had become constantly tired. From long experience, I suggested that his metabolism might have altered during the years, making 60 grams of carbohydrate either too much or, more likely, too little. He quickly learned that the fatigue disappeared when he added half of a baked potato at two meals daily, and optimal well-being returned.

In closing our discussion of the mischief makers, sugars and starches, let me give you some sources of information that will help you, after the preliminary testing, to fix accurately the carbohydrate level in your diet. One of them lists the carbohydrate and calorie values of most common foods: *Carlton Fredericks' Calorie and Carbohydrate Guide,* a paperback published by Pocket Books. From the same publisher, giving instruction in the use of bran, an important addition to a low-carbohydrate diet, is *Carlton Fredericks' High-Fiber Way to Total Health*. Low-carbohydrate menus, at the approximate 60-gram level, will be found in my *Low Blood Sugar and You* paperback, published by Grosset and Dunlap. *Don't* try to use these texts for the bases of an optimal carbohydrate intake without the preliminary testing just described. They're not intended for that purpose.

FAT REQUIREMENT TESTING

The fat requirement presents even knottier technical problems, involving not only the kind of fat—saturated or polyunsaturated (vegetable oil)—but also the amounts. With vegetable oils, there is an amount set by the need for weight loss, and another ceiling, for those who need not reduce, set by prudence, for excessive intake of polyunsaturated fat can be dangerous. Overheated, these oils can be carcinogenic. In excessive amounts, you have already learned, they can cause premature aging. In any case, they increase your need for the antioxidants which help to retard aging. I limit the polyunsaturated fats to no more than 20 percent of the total fat intake, which in the average American diet is about 35 percent. If I have not already dissuaded you from worrying about the effects of saturated fats in raising blood cholesterol, or pledging your faith in the cholesterol-lowering actions claimed for vegetable oil, let me tell you flatly that the disappointing results from applying this philosophy to the prevention of cardiovascular disease could have been predicted. Cholesterol elevation is not a disease, but a symptom, and one doesn't treat symptoms. Every medical student is taught that symptomatic medicine is bad medicine, but doesn't learn that elevated blood cholesterol is but the iceberg's tip, and underneath there is the real mischief maker: stress. Do you think the elevated blood cholesterol in medical students at examination time and in accountants at tax time is a coincidence? All this means that the claims made for vegetable oils are sheer advertising puffery, and dangerous, at that. You will not only be cheated of the promised protection against cardiovascular disorders, but you will run a distinctly increased risk of cancer and premature old age.

The blood chemistries I have described will give your medical nutritionist clues to your fat tolerance and utilization, and thereby to the type and amount you should be eating, and the supplements you should be taking. The antioxidants are useful to anyone, but some of us will need help in fat-utilization and metabolism. For example, there are nutrients that not only help to regulate blood cholesterol levels, but also raise the blood content of the type of cholesterol (high-density lipoprotein) that is protective, rather than harmful. Among these, as examples, are vitamin E and lecithin, which you should be using anyway for their antioxidant effects.

With stress as a prime mover behind elevations in blood fats which may sometimes be inappropriate responses by the body, alteration of life-style becomes imperative. If your medical practitioner does not feel competent to supervise such needed changes, he may refer you to a psychologist or psychiatrist. Don't ignore the recommendation, which may be more vital than you realize. For example, I have mentioned that "Type A" personalities—perfectionists, trying to do two things at once, always racing with the clock— are at greater risk of heart attacks than the rest of us. What do you think happens when a man who is Type A marries a woman who also is? Answer: his risk of heart attack goes up by a factor of *six*. It suggests that a Type A man who marries a non-Type-A woman should expect his wedding expenses to be paid by medical insurance. It also tells you that cholesterol levels in the blood are but a facet of a multi-ordinate equation, not to be solved by restriction of eggs or swigging of vegetable oils.

Along with your glucose tolerance test, then, your physician will appraise blood cholesterol, levels of high-density and low-density lipoproteins, triglycerides,* uric acid, and adhesiveness of blood platelets. The results will determine whether the antioxidants you use to combat aging will play a double role, in helping to keep arteries and heart healthy. They will also indicate whether you should be supplementing your diet with concentrated fish oils, or eating more oily fish.

If all this sounds costly and time-consuming, it is. But let me remind you: when a degenerative disease strikes, and your doctor gives you the diagnosis, one of your early questions will be: "What should I eat?" Ask it *now*.

Without knowledge of these blood chemistries, every meal you eat is a voyage into the unknown. This much we know: if my readers are American adults, we can make a firm prophecy: one in three of you, at the age of sixty-five, *will* have a degenerative disease. Not only are such disorders less common in the well-nourished, but for the large majority of them, medicine has no cures. How many times have you heard a physician say: "You have arthritis; take aspirin and learn to live with it"?

Books that offer a single system of diet as *the* diet for every reader are frequently best-sellers. Yet every nutritionist worthy of the title knows that Jack Spratt exists, and so does his wife. Interestingly, the Spratts at this minute are sharing exactly the same menus.

VITAMIN REQUIREMENT TESTING

While there are health professionals who rely on tests of vitamin blood levels, most of us recognize them as yielding largely meaningless results. There are two reasons (now familiar to you) for this, the first being that the body compensates for low blood levels by moving into the blood vitamin supplies from the tissues, in an obvious effort to distribute a limited, vital resource more equitably. The second reason involves enzymes, of which many vitamins and some minerals are components. If the enzyme is the form in which

---

*Excessive sugar intake for some people is the route to elevated triglycerides.

the vitamin is utilized, the level of the vitamin in the blood is academic. This is parallel to what we have learned about vitamin C. Blood levels of ascorbic acid don't tell us whether the vitamin has been efficiently put to use in the white cells and in the tissues; and we have tests for these, which are thereby much more meaningful than the level of ascorbic acid in the blood.

If we find that adding the vitamin to a sample of your blood raises the level of the enzyme in which it is a component, it indicates that you may have a need for higher intake of that nutrient, and satisfying it will offer a potential for better health and added longevity. If you don't respond to the vitamin by increasing your enzyme level, it may indicate that your intake is already optimal, or it may point to a block in the biochemical pathway by which a vitamin becomes part of an enzyme. To a limited extent, these blockade points can sometimes be detoured. At any rate, for a number of vitamins, these tests can give important clues to individual differences in vitamin needs. In some cases, though, administration of these nutrients by mouth may not yield the anticipated dividends. This points to a problem in utilization and absorption of the factors, inviting examination for adequacy of digestive function or the presence of conditions leading to malabsorption. All these findings are invaluable in helping to satisfy your unique nutritional requirements.

MINERAL REQUIREMENT TESTING

As it can with vitamins, the body will shift minerals from the tissues when supplies are short, making blood levels and hair levels of minerals unreliable guides to the adequacy of intake and efficiency of utilization of minerals. Certain enzyme tests are helpful, since metals, zinc and copper being good examples, participate in a large number of enzyme chemistries. Combined analyses of blood, urine, and hair levels may also yield more meaningful information. Though hair analysis has been criticized by ignorant professions, the fact is that while it alone should not be the basis for decision about dietary needs, it does constitute a record of past months, while blood and urine largely speak for today only. This tells you that recommendation of vitamin-mineral supplements on the basis of hair analysis is a serious error. At the same time, it is sometimes vital to life itself to appraise the body's levels of the minerals that are components of enzyme systems. As an example, low levels of selenium in the blood will inhibit an enzyme system vital to slowing the aging process and to raising resistance of women to breast cancer and of men to heart disease.

We are gradually arriving at workable norms (ranges) for blood, urine, and hair content of essential minerals and metals. Your medical nutritionist has access to laboratories where such determinations are made. The corrective procedure goes in both directions: raising the levels of those essential nutrients which are too low, and bringing down those which are too high. In the latter classification, there are some invaders of the body that in any amount are threatening. These are the heavy metals, and as you read the next paragraph, don't assume that it applies to someone else. You would be startled by the number of people we find whose bodies harbor, without their knowledge, levels of heavy metals that threaten the nervous system and the brain.

Both blood and hair levels of heavy metals will be appraised, for the obvious reason that health is threatened by accumulations of lead, mercury, and cadmium, even in what would seem to be low levels. For example, the levels of lead in the blood of children have been linked with subtle neurological disorders and learning difficulties, even in quantities that a few years ago were considered innocuous. The potential of mercury for mischief is brought to mind by the Mad Hatter, who was the victim of the mercury used in the manufacture of felt for hats. Cadmium is indicted for kidney disease linked with high blood pressure. Excesses of copper and iron are a threat, too. Those exposed to these metals in their occupation—the thermometer maker, the foundry employee—are not the only ones at risk, for we find undesirably high levels of toxic metals in individuals whose exposure was not industrial, and remains conjectural. At any rate, there are nutritional therapies for some of these conditions, and chelation, recommended earlier for atherosclerosis, was originally employed for lead poisoning, and still is. Aluminum is another threat, linked with an early type of senility with brain damage, marked by high concentrations of the metal in nerve fibers. This is problematical, for there are those with high aluminum levels who remain normal, but we have as yet no way to appraise the risk to which they are exposed. You acquire aluminum,

I might mention, not only from its use in clarifying drinking water, but in many antacid drugs, from possible absorption from the use of deodorants, from baking powder, and many other sources. The chelating agent used for excessive iron levels—deferoxamine—is also believed to remove aluminum. A number of dietary constituents, among them the "trace" minerals, offer some protection against toxic metal accumulation. This makes zinc and calcium intake, among others, even more important to you, as well as magnesium and manganese.

PROTEIN REQUIREMENTS

Endless filing cabinets are filled with slander of high-protein diets. A half-century ago, vegetarians were assuring anyone who would listen that animal protein causes everything from kidney troubles to hypertension and cancer. They weren't silenced when an Arctic explorer and his associate, under the scrutiny of physicians at Bellevue Hospital in New York City, lived on meat and fat alone, for a year, and emerged healthier on this Eskimo-type diet than they had been when the experiment started. Though dire warnings are issued about the adverse effects of high protein intake, to this day, one of my former students has achieved remarkable results in the physical and mental rejuvenation of fading movie stars, using a regimen of *400 grams* of animal protein daily, coupled with exercise and massage. The gloomy prophecies ignore an ancient axiom: the food most efficient for a given species is that which most closely resembles the composition of the species. We aren't made of cornflakes. Moreover, the animals that violate this tenet, such as the horse and the cow, must spend hours in filling their stomachs. Creatures so constituted and so fed would have had no time to acquire intelligence, build a culture, and pass their wisdom on to their posterity. Particularly obnoxious, scientifically, are the eulogies of peas, beans, and high-carbohydrate diets, which, we are told, will make us immune to a long list of degenerative diseases—to which vegetarian animals aren't immune. While carbohydrate tolerances, as you have read, vary widely, and some individuals thrive on a high intake of complex carbohydrates, no one escapes the need for an adequate supply of efficient protein, and contrary to the vegetarian legends about soy, other legumes, and vegetable proteins, none of these is as complete and efficient in meeting human needs as the protein derived from animal sources. Moreover, there is no scheme of diet and no food supplements which will be effective in the absence of any essential amino (protein) acid from the daily food intake. The body is unprepared for such deficiency, and reacts to inadequate intake of a single amino acid as if *all* amino acids were missing. It is because of this phenomenon that I have likened nutrition to a fabric of many threads.

Should you be slated for surgery, or relegated to a hospital intensive-care unit, the content of the blood in two protein factors will give us a firm basis for estimating your chances for complications and, indeed, survival. There is a fourfold increase in complications and a sixfold increase in deaths when the blood albumin level is at or below 3.5 grams per deciliter. Deaths are *twenty* times as frequent when the total white cell count is less than 1,500 per cubic millimeter. This kind of arithmetic becomes even more relentless in patients placed in intensive-care units of hospitals. Here low levels in these factors were six to eleven times more frequent than in those patients not requiring such close monitoring—meaning that they were less sick. Not only do you bring yesterday's and yesteryear's menus with you when you are hospitalized, but these figures trace a direct relationship between your protein intake and your chances of living to a ripe old age.

With all this, protein foods are the most costly in the diet, and despite the high level of "average American" protein consumption, inadequate intake is common. Averages are deceptive, for they represent a figure above and below which the majority of the population may fall.

The problem may be aggravated by malutilization, because of lack of a vitamin, a digestive enzyme, an enzyme needed in metabolism, or stomach hydrochloric acid. It is academic whether a nutrient such as protein is inadequately supplied by the diet or inefficiently utilized by the body; the net effect will be malnutrition with your stomach well filled, a prescription for illness and premature aging.

Protein requirements are sometimes determined, if that word doesn't create an illusion, by ascertaining the amount of such foods necessary to prevent negative nitrogen balance. The vegetarians and the Pritikins have a love affair with that concept, for it brings the need for protein to an absolute minimum. Essentially, what is being measured is the lowest amount of protein that will keep the body from raiding its own tissues. This is analogous to setting the vitamin C requirement at the daily 10-mg. dose needed to prevent scurvy. As we know that intake beyond that level yields dividends, so do we know that the absolute minimum level of protein doesn't pave the way to optimal health. A more reasonable amount is suggested by more valid research, which sets the adult protein requirement at about one-half gram per pound of normal body weight. Thus a man weighing 160 pounds would require about 80 grams of protein daily. Not all of this would come from animal proteins, but they are the most efficient. Less efficient proteins, such as those supplied by beans, peas, other legumes, and whole grains, will become more valuable if served at the same meal with protein of animal origin. Thus your meat makes the protein of the peas and potato more adequate. All this is simply an example of an amino acid, missing from or inadequately supplied by one food, being supplied from another, better protein. This action requires that the foods which will complement each other be taken at the same meal. Those with a limited budget, therefore, fare better if the limited amount of animal protein they can afford is divided among the day's meals, rather than served in one portion.

On the basis of very limited research with a few animals and human subjects, the statement is made that a high-protein diet, defined as more than 90 grams of protein daily, causes excretion of needed minerals. This conclusion means that the far North should be littered with Eskimos whose skeletons have given way, and that the Masai, whose diet is crammed with protein, should likewise be a vanished race. In those individuals who need and poorly tolerate high protein intake, the obvious answer is the use of a supplement of multiple minerals, the potency determined by the degree of excretion.

There is a formidable amount of evidence that the cooking of protein foods as we commonly practice it with meat, fish, fowl, eggs, and the pasteurization of milk and cheese alters the foods subtly, so that they do not properly support reproduction. The impact is on the pituitary (actually, the anterior pituitary) of the young. Some uncooked protein in the diet, at least in pregnancy, would be an investment in caution. At any rate, the next time you read that high-protein nutrition is a menace to man, keep his history in mind. He was for millennia on the hunter-herdsman's diet, and survived well enough to perpetuate the race. Nor did that diet impair his ability to initiate and preserve his culture. Isn't it food for thought to realize that no vegetarian people has ever made a significant contribution to that culture?

None of this denies that there are those who function better on lower protein and more of the complex carbohydrates. They serve to remind us that the only permissible generalization about dietary needs is the fact that no generalizations are possible.

CHOOSING YOUR SUPPLEMENTS

I have already emphasized that supplements must not be used as a license for eating junk food or an unbalanced diet. The purpose of these concentrates is double: dietary insurance, certainly sensible in the absence of definite information about the nutrient content of your diet; and higher intake than you could achieve from food, without gaining excess weight.

The basic supplement is a multiple vitamin, multiple mineral concentrate. Chelated minerals are more costly and with a few exceptions (copper among them) offer no advantage for a healthy person with a normal digestive tract. Don't choose a vitamin-mineral concentrate on the basis of a long and imposing list of nutrients. Many such products have insignificant amounts of some of the factors, making the label impressive for the nutritionally unsophisticated. With the multiple vitamin-mineral concentrate, a separate, natural source of the vitamin B complex should be used. The most easily available would be, in the order of preference, desiccated liver, brewer's yeast, and wheat germ. The liver capsules or tablets should, preferably, be derived from Argentine sources, to avoid the concentration of insecticides or hormones, or both, which appear in some batches of American origin; though it should be noted that this doesn't occur regularly, and the concentration is minor. Those allergic to liver may be able to tolerate brewer's yeast, though that, too, contains many (fifty) substances to which a person might be sensitive or allergic. Dosage is not critical, for these are foods, but to explore tolerance, observe the ancient rule "Little dose, little allergy," and start with minimum amounts, working your way up. This is the same technique recommended for bran, if you recall. Wheat germ is unlikely to cause an intestinal uproar, unless you're allergic to wheat, but small initial quantities, added to cereal or used as a cereal, will explore that. Wheat germ may also be added to flour, one teaspoonful per cup of flour, offering excellent added nutritional values, including important antioxidants. If there is a history in your family of schizophrenia or celiac disease, both wheat germ and wheat may be as undesirable for you as it is for sufferers of multiple sclerosis. A handful of liver tablets or brewer's yeast tablets is your ultimate goal, but you start with one or two tablets and sample your gastrointestinal climate.

The fat-soluble vitamins are usually supplied by the multiple vitamin concentrate, but—usually, again—some of them are inadequately represented. The optimal intake of vitamin A, to meet the actual range of needs, may be between 5,000 and 33,000 units daily for adults. An average supplement provides 10,000 units. Some people, obviously, will profit by more. Pro-vitamin-A, which is beta carotene, now identified with resistance to cancer as well as antioxidant effects, is also available in supplements and can be used with your vitamin A concentrate. From 10,000 to 25,000 units daily would be reasonable. Oddly, though carotene is converted in the body to vitamin A (except in diabetics), none of the toxic reactions attributed to vitamin A are found with beta carotene, except for tinting the skin yellow if you overdo it.

Vitamin D, normally obtained through the action of sunlight on the skin, is provided adequately by the average multiple supplement. Overdose is possible; in fact, the numerous sources of vitamin D_3 in the diet, particularly in milk products, has been suspected of causing arthritic changes in individuals sensitive to it. If you live in the Sun Belt, your vitamin D is free, and that in the supplement will be a reasonable addition.

Vitamin K, known as the blood-clotting vitamin, is not available without a prescription, for the good reason that excessive clotting is much more frequent a tendency than hemorrhaging. However, vitamin K has an important role in calcium metabolism, which I find seldom recognized, and for women and older men who want to avoid osteoporosis, the use of green vegetables or their juice will be a reasonable source of this vitamin.

The vitamin E content of the average multiple supplement is quantitatively unsatisfactory, and so is the form of the vitamin, usually alpha tocopherol. You now know that you want *mixed* tocopherols, meaning alpha, beta, gamma, and delta forms, because this is the way you obtain maximum antioxidant effects. One uses mixed tocopherol capsules, augmenting the small amount in the multiple supplement, in potencies of 200 to 400 units. These are not the medicinal doses, which may be much higher in phlebitis and intermittent claudication, among other disorders. Do not accept any vitamin E with the prefix *dl*. This is synthetic, and less desirable than mixed tocopherols.

Zinc is used in the form of the gluconate, which is less costly than chelated zinc, and as well utilized. Supplementary amounts, including whatever zinc content is in the multiple mineral supplement, can be 15 to 30 mg. daily. If you are a male troubled with an enlarged prostate, your medical nutritionist will prescribe much higher potencies. Copper, on the other hand, is often toxic in the inorganic form, and is best used as a chelate. A safe amount is 2 mg. daily, unless you live in an area with soft water and copper plumbing. Higher doses of the metal, which sometimes are important therapeutically, require monitoring of blood and hair levels.

Octocosanol, the energy factor in wheat, is a normal constituent of the oil in wheat germ. When used in the concentrated form as a supplement, it is best taken in capsules containing the nutrient in concentrated wheat germ oil, for this will provide other "waxy alcohols" that normally accompany octocosanol and have physiological activity. The lowest potency available is 375 mcg., roughly one-third of a milligram, and one to three capsules daily are used. For those who want higher potencies for reduced dosage of the supplement, there are similar products containing 2 mg. per capsule.

Marine lipid concentrates, used to normalize blood cholesterol and triglycerides, and to reduce the viscosity of blood and the adhesiveness of blood platelets, are available in capsules containing a significant concentration of the fatty acids that have these effects. The label dosage, usually one or two capsules daily, is a worthwhile supplementation. Medically, they may be administered literally by the dozens, something you do not try on your own.

Selenium, best used in the bound form, which means concentrated in a special yeast, is used in potencies of 50 mcg. I know there are texts that suggest much more. I also know that some people experience toxic effects at these high levels. We consume about 200 mcg. in our daily food, if well selected, while the Japanese, largely because of their fish intake, have about 500 mcg. daily. Thus, 50 mcg. seems a reasonable protective amount, considering that the nutrient may help to protect women, as it does Japanese women, against cancer, and men against one type of heart disease. You need the selenium for another reason: it is an activator of the vitamin E you will be taking.

Choline may be included in the multiple supplement, but usually not in rewarding quantities. One may take choline as such, or combined in a tablet with inositol. For women, to invoke protection against estrogens, whether internally produced or prescribed by the physician, the potencies should be 1,000 mg. of choline and 500 mg. of inositol. In trying to help cognition and memory in the aged, these quantities are often doubled. Choline may also be taken in the form of lecithin. If you are using lecithin granules, probably the most inexpensive form, two tablespoonfuls daily would be a good investment. In capsules, this quantity would be too difficult to achieve, unless you choose the high phosphatidyl choline lecithin products, which, being three times as potent in choline as ordinary lecithin, can be used in small amounts. In addition to the favorable effects of lecithin on blood fats and in increasing high-density lipoprotein, it is, of course, often used to help circulation and mental function in the aged and senile.

Tryptophane is used in quantities between 500 and 1,500 mg. for the purpose of shortening sleep latency. Enormously greater amounts are used therapeutically, in Parkinson's disease, but that requires additional phenylalanine, and needs medical supervision. Tryptophane in similar supplementary quantities is also used to help the depressed and, combined with vitamin B_6 and niacinamide supplements, to treat obsessive-compulsive behavior.

Vitamin B_{12}, alone or combined with folic acid, is used in the form of lozenges that are absorbed by placing them under the tongue. Potency varies from 500 to 1,000 mcg. of B_{12} per lozenge, and from 400 mcg. to 1 mg. of folic acid.

The quantity of vitamins B_1 and B_2 (thiamine and riboflavin) in the multiple vitamin supplement should be adequate for the average user. When there is a higher requirement, the so-called "50-50-50" formulas are helpful. The quantities refer to B_1, B_2, and niacinamide. Niacinamide, though, when used to help prevent arthritic changes, is needed in larger amounts, as high as 1 gram (1,000 mg.) daily. Niacin, the form of the vitamin that induces a flush, is best used in time-release form. Only experience will tell what potency best suits the user, but from 100 to 200 mg. daily, in time-release form, would be a good compromise for many users.

Inositol, which I use with choline to help women with estrogen-dependent disorders such as cystic breast disease, menstrual disturbances, endometriosis, and uterine fibroid tumors, is usually employed in 500-mg. potency, as I have indicated. Sometimes, though, this nutrient has a remarkable "tranquilizer" effect, and for that purpose, the potency is raised to one gram (1,000 mg) daily. Taken at the hour of sleep, together with tryptophane, inositol helps in achieving more restful sleep for some individuals. It also helps diabetics with problems in nerve function.

Calcium pantothenate, used to help adrenal function, and in the treatment of rheumatoid arthritis, senility, and gastric ulcer, is employed in potencies of 750 mg. to 1 gram (1,000 mg.) daily.

Vitamin C, which I personally use in time-release form, is available in that form in potencies of 500 and 1,500 mg. per tablet. These are used morning and night. Some individuals profit by more, and I have already indicated that Dr. Linus Pauling estimates actual needs to range from 250 mg. to 2,500 daily. There *are* dividends from intake far beyond the modest estimates of the conservative authorities.

My personal intake of PABA is 1,000 mg. daily. This, however, is in a prescription form (potassium salt of PABA), which dissolves more readily than PABA as it is sold commercially, and therefore is equivalent to more than a gram of ordinary PABA. For many individuals, the range of profitable intake would be from 100 to 500 mg. daily.

The bioflavonoids, preferably of citrus origin, are used in 1 gram potency for supplements. Therapeutic doses are much higher. It is as important to use the bioflavonoids as it is to use concentrated vitamin C, which, incidentally, the bioflavonoids protect against oxidation in the body. Rutin is not recommended.

The pyridoxine (vitamin B_6) content of the average multiple supplement is adequate for many users. However, there are circumstances where the need is higher. Large intake of niacinamide raises pyridoxine needs. So does the presence of the Chinese restaurant syndrome or carpal tunnel syndrome, or certain cases of arthritis, or premenstrual water retention. In such instances, the B_6 intake required may rise as high as 250 mg. daily; it is even higher in some autistic children and in a type of schizophrenia.

RNA, the memory molecule—and remember not to use it if you have elevated uric acid or an actual case of gout—is taken in quantities up to 2 grams daily.

Finally, while I prefer to obtain protein from succulent sources like good food, there are sometimes problems with utilization or allergy that can be solved by administration of combinations of essential amino acids for sublingual (under the tongue) administration, which permits direct absorption, bypassing the digestive tract. This solves severe problems for some troubled people.

SAFETY NOTES

Anyone can be allergic to or intolerant of *anything*. If you don't tolerate a vitamin, mineral, or protein, or react adversely to, say, marine oils, make sure that you are in fact intolerant of the nutrient, for it may be a filler, excipient, coloring agent, or preservative that is insulting your interior. There are brands of supplements that specifically omit such extraneous ingredients. You are safer with these.

Supplements for pregnant women are a breed apart. An expectant mother should not follow these recommendations. The diet and supplements in pregnancy, well tested by decades of experience, are in my *Nutrition Handbook,* available in paperback.

Note that supplements provide factors usually found in food, and should be taken *with* food, whether before or after a meal. Other than tryptophane and inositol, supplements are best taken early in the day. There is no esoteric reason for this; it is merely that the concentrates are often stimulating, which is fine in relieving fatigue, but unhappy when you're trying to go to sleep.

Patience is a vitamin, too, which must be taken with the good basic diet and the supplements. Nutritional responses don't share the "miracle drug" mystique. Time is of the essence, and many failures to achieve maximum benefits come from short-term trials of what should be a lifetime program. I wish you from application of these nutritional data the same dividends which came to me, over a long lifetime.

Index